Mental Models

Improving Productivity, Decision Making Skills and Critical Thinking Mechanism

(Mental Training to Improve Focus and Self-discipline)

Jason Nelson

I0106000

Published By **Jackson Denver**

Jason Nelson

Mental Models: Improving Productivity, Decision Making Skills and Critical Thinking Mechanism (Mental Training to Improve Focus and Self-discipline)

ISBN   978-1-998769-99-5

No part of this guidebook shall be reproduced in any form without permission in writing from the publisher except in the case of brief quotations embodied in critical articles or reviews.

Legal & Disclaimer

The information contained in this ebook is not designed to replace or take the place of any form of medicine or professional medical advice. The information in this ebook has been provided for educational & entertainment purposes only.

The information contained in this book has been compiled from sources deemed reliable, and it is accurate to the best of the Author's knowledge; however, the Author cannot guarantee its accuracy and validity and cannot be held liable for any errors or omissions. Changes are periodically made to this book. You must consult your doctor or get professional medical advice before using any of the suggested remedies, techniques, or information in this book.

Table of Contents

Introduction

Do you ever experience trapped in your personal head? Maybe you're looking to clear up a hassle or understand why someone acts a certain manner, but you keep going around in a circle. You recognize a specific angle could help, or searching at things from a special attitude, but you aren't sure how to get there. Enter mental models.

Mental fashions are like gear in a toolbox. They every have a particular cause and layout, and are acceptable to different tasks. The more mental fashions you have for your psychological toolbox, the more types of questioning tasks you can tackle. If you just had one tool, your effectiveness and mental talents would be very limited. Have you ever attempted sawing a bit of wood with a hammer? It doesn't work.

There's any other assessment we are able to make with mental models: digital camera lenses. Camera lenses can help you see the same view (like a sunrise or mountain or cityscape) in a myriad of different ways. A fisheye lens offers you a absolutely wide perspective, even as a zooming lens lets you get in the direction of specific gadgets inside the view. The extra mental lenses you've got, the more information and clarity you may get on a situation or hassle.

In this book, you'll be added to the extensive world of intellectual models and the way they could practice to each area of your existence, whether it's selection-making, trouble-fixing, seeing matters extra virtually, navigating relationships, or questioning more undoubtedly. While they'll seem complex at first look, incorporating greater mental models in your life definitely makes a lot of sense, and lots of them would possibly already be a every day practice for you. This ebook gives them names and clearer definitions, so you can be more intentional about expanding your questioning and perspectives.

Chapter 1: Understanding Your Mental Model

There are quite many reasons for warfare even though they sooner or later can be distilled into the fact that we've numerous intellectual fashions of the way the planet works. The intellectual fashions are either hurtful or beneficial.

On the only hand, they may be extremely beneficial in how they guard us and simplify our lives from the strength of being compelled to reconsider each view we have each time we're faced with a scenario.

These designs tend to be contextual. We have various variations for every facet of every day lifestyles, from who we pick out to be buddies with, to what track type we be aware of, to the sorts of meals we devour, and the make of car we pressure.

Your parameters and mental model for eating place selection might be the restaurant use domestically grown produce and have a vegetarian choice in large part at reasonable fees. Your pal can also have a intellectual design that dictates they dine in highly-priced restaurants with the best wines and most useful cuts of red meat.

These are the complete opposite ends of the spectrum, and consequently there isn't a whole lot of a compromise for the folks in a single or the other stop at discovering a place they can dine together (i.E., the financial element by using itself is, in essence, a deal-breaker while neither is prepared to budge).

Or take, as an example, your desire in where you reside. One man or woman needs to dwell in a metropolitan area surrounded through exercise, galleries, eating places, theater, shops, and variety, and their associate desires to stay in a small or rural t surroundings where there's garden among the houses and one-forestall sign in the town.

We do not understand purposely that those intellectual fashions might be in movement up until we come up towards someone who has opposite intellectual models. If you're among like-minded individuals in an isolated surroundings, you may surely live away from the expertise of in my opinion know-how other versions of the arena are practicable.

It isn't always that you do no longer understand those different values are out there; nonetheless, since you apprehend versions of believe are available at the least based totally on television, films, and the web.

Problems stand up whilst we aren't aware of our intellectual models. We can get caught and be stubborn and believe ours will be the only manner. I actually have observed this arise with more mature human beings in my family -- there are a right way and a wrong manner, so this is how it is.

They trust that there may be one strategy for the arena to do the process, and the troubles of the arena lay inside the noncompliance of every body who does now not percentage their world view.

That is probably a remarkably huge burden to turn out to be the keeper of the fact concerning the manner the sector works. How does this fit into persuasion?

Effectively, that falls under the heading of knowledge thyself. When we excavate our intellectual fashions, we are able to overturn engineer where matters are not working, or if they're operating, we will opposite engineer to decide how we've end up very effective at what we take place.

Are Your Mental Models On The Low Or High Road?

Mental variations will be described as "generalizations, deeply ingrained assumptions, and pics of pictures that have an effect on how we convey an movement and recognize the world."

Mental models do have a sizeable impact on how we see, reply to, and react to the sector; they situation our satisfactory-of-existence, relationships, and decisions. They have an effect on us on almost all tiers - private, organizational, expert, social, global, and national.

My motive is raising your degree of understanding of what intellectual models are and the manner they perform. Useful neuroscience standards and tools assist you to challenge, trade, and control your mental models for a higher, more non violent, and less stressful existence.

Private Observations

☐ Mental models are saved data and mental imprints of the way your thoughts perceived and remembered instant man or woman reports and data learned from a third birthday party or indirect tool which includes the clicking.

☐ Models on the way to yield harmful outcomes for you and others are extraordinary candidates for exam and altered questioning.

☐ Formed over the years from amassed info, they might be created deeply and quick based totally on their significance and mental impact.

☐ Most individuals are blind to their fashions, wherever they got here from, and their results.

☐ They are challenging and diffused to pick out and describe.

☐ They appear to run in a "backroom" or unconscious a part of our brain.

☐ Our fashions regularly get more potent with time as human nature would like to be "proper" regarding their critiques.

☐ They may also or might not be verifiable through impartial observations or direct enjoy from integrous human beings.

I think the center issue is "how rightly do the intellectual models paintings me and others," as opposed to "are my intellectual variations suitable or incorrect?" There is no right way of consuming and processing sensory info because absolutely everyone perceives and interprets info in a different way.

A group of people agreeing on one thing does now not make it actual; the manner binds the group around what they preserve to be real. Needless arguments and wars occur because of versions of opinion regarding mental models.

Evaluating

These each day life conditions provide you with a hold close of what intellectual fashions appear like; every pair has versions of mindset for illustrative functions. As you appearance them over, reflect onconsideration on which ones may also serve you and a few first-rate, rather of selecting what might be accurate or in mistakes.

The goal of this workout is shifting your cognizance to a "high street" or a terrific perspective for comparing mental fashions. With success, those examples will stimulate your thinking to jot down down the mental models that serve you poorly or properly.

Minimal Road: Good thoughts for improvement are drying up, and there may be a constrained commercial enterprise opportunity for me to prosper.

High Road: Good thoughts for brand new merchandise, technology, and services are infinite and endless.

_____

—

_____

—

_____

—

Low Road: We are now residing in a competitive global of scarcity.

Great Road: We are actually residing in a global of boundless possibility in which by situational cooperation is doable.

_____

—

_____

—

_____

—

Low Road: Girls do badly on science and math.

Higher Road: Anyone can find out what pastimes her or him, whilst in a supportive surroundings.

_____

____

_____

____

_____

____

Low Road: You can't believe in who appear like, act and speak a specific way.

Higher Road: There are untrustworthy and truthful individuals in all areas of lifestyles.

_____

____

_____

____

_____

____

Low Road: In this monetary system, nobody will interview me, lots less, rent me.

Great Road: I even have tremendous trends and transferable abilities that some organization is attempting to find.

_____

____

_____

____

_____

____

Low Road: I cannot agree with in myself behind the controls because of my using document and even what my partner says.

Higher Road: A renewal route will make me a greater secure, more reliable and a ways better shielding driver.

_____

____

_____

____

_____

___

Low Road: I can not examine things that are new because I created bad grades and my teacher stated I turned into dumb.

High Road: My brain has limitless capability to develop, get more potent, taken into consideration rapid and make brilliant choices.

_____

___

_____

___

_____

___

Low Road: It isn't probable I will live past seventy three because of my own family health history.

High Road: A wholesome frame practices and an optimistic mental mindset will growth my satisfactory-of-existence and perhaps add years to my life span.

Mental fashions are what we feel and preserve to be correct about existence. They are our "software programming" that drives questioning, behaviors, and reviews. There is normally an outcome from each mental version, even though they might not be apparent. Individuals vehemently agree and disagree on the truth in their mental models.

The defining moment for challenging a intellectual version happens as soon as the emphasis shifts to the favored result. Clarity can great be performed by way of analyzing gaps among what's desired and the outcome that occurs. This is the only way I know breaking the endless cycle of shielding and attacking mental fashions.

Effects Of Thinking Pattern On Life

The concept and that means of existence are charming subjects of dialogue. How we view it, on the begin, is an area to contemplate. What is becoming transpired and conspired, after delivery to the give up, is the passage, we revel in in multi-dimensional mode. The multitude and variance of thoughts replicate a large amount of people's heads and their wondering styles.

The significance of life is a philosophical entity in the idea of performance and existence. Our life of duty is immediately proportional to our expectations and commitments. We are had to meet obligations inside the ambit of dos and don'ts.

You will discover rules, guidelines, and pointers imposed on human beings as soon as we accept our realities and existence. There isn't any room for hypothetical deductions or fantasies. On the other hand, records and factuality are existence design. The life span goes in a way as created with the aid of us.

The creational fact comprehensively balances between effect and reason. A unique takes its lead from information and understanding, a gift from the author. Today, the motion and response reflect an person's thinking layout.

It adversely impacts are encountered through individuals even as inside the passage of existence span. It leaves its sizable effects sincerely and particularly. Nevertheless, few apprehend its implication, and some forget about it. A question comes up regarding the reason these anomalies surface whilst realities are open, and factuality seemed?

When specifics and phenomenon are open, a person or group ignores it despite enough proof, in the end boastful sets in. Consequently, all the ill consequences appear as useful and superb. Hence, they get taken away into chaos and commotion, accepting the useful realities.

Thus, the wondering layout of a non-public dictates its phrases and compels her or him to renowned the influence as realities. This is an critical reputation, and one must exercise warning and get the utmost care. If he or she succeeds, therefore, experiencing contentment and bliss.

The after-effect of the collection of thinking shows and advises that evaluating the hassle need to be the priority. You will discover some smart males that assume twice earlier than creating a choice and react.

The crucial point of the matter can be the end result of ideas, and they are a center factor of the layout of wondering. At this factor, the reactionary forces may produce hurdles that have an effect on the form of questioning; for this reason, it impacts our life in a different way.

The truth is based on the realities of residing as experienced through parents they be given it. The denial can be the negativity and stubbornness of a person intentionally relegating factuality and statistics. Thus, the thinking layout of someone is ruled with the aid of two factors.

The simple path of fact leaves an wonderful effect on the lifestyles of a person. On the flip aspect, an boastful individual's line of questioning and method is grounded on deception and falsehood. He prospers on fantasies and gets into myth.

The crux of the topic is the development of thoughts allowing a ordinary man or woman to take manage line of questioning. It usually prospers on some essential troubles of cognition, emotions, or violation and feelings. Individuals after which get affected correctly situation to environments and conditions. They consider that things are designed to in shape their goals.

They behave violently when encountering screw ups or denial. These are the peripheral perceptional dispositions. Nevertheless, a person other than a everyday character will react differently due to the capability to evaluate and observe the state of affairs in actualities and realities. He views outside of the horizon and appreciates the unexpected and seen results in real phrases relegating fantasies at the back of.

Chapter 2: What Are Mental Models And Why Are They Important?

Usually, people gather the capability to assume from the reflection of shared recognition in the community. When every person round you may receive the shared reflection of awareness, you may now not feel to elevate any doubt about it. Mental models involve ideas, classifications, characteristics, prototype and stereotype descriptions, world views, and regular narration. Most of the decisions taken via the people inside their normal life are based at the standards of mental models. Without the life of intellectual models, there are such a lot of activities along with information to each different, getting answers for the issues regards to behave collectively, a feeling of sensitivity for belonging and solidarity and development of an organization for the welfare of the society.

Definition of Mental Models

People receive thoughts, faiths, pictures and verbal explanations consciously or unconsciously from their experience. Mental models are a representation of recognized reality with the reason of motive and bring about the surroundings. They lead the humans to maintain expectation for gaining certain effects and additionally permit to apprehend the which means of the occasions and even to predispose people to conduct in positive approaches. You can evaluate mental fashions to an architectural structure's blueprint. A blueprint is a short description of the ability structure that can be built doubtlessly within the actual global. Mental fashions are just like a blueprint of an architectural structure describing reasonable opportunities of events that exist inside the real global.

Mental fashions are the starting factors for all styles of reasoning tactics. Mental models are crucial as they've some specific identities. Some of the unique identities of intellectual models are as follows:

·Mental models aren't finished as there growing continuously new styles of conditions and troubles in the real international. So, humans are used to coping up with this changeable state of affairs and problems by using evolving numerous types of intellectual fashions continually.

·Sometimes, mental models are did not describe accurately an event and then the simple principle of models is not correct and additionally includes contradictions.

·Mental models provide brief and simplified descriptions of a complicated occasion. Then, human beings can without problems realize and get the solution effortlessly for a complex trouble of their existence.

·There are several conditions and action policies are taken into consideration while one of the unique intellectual models represents the descriptions.

Mental fashions assist to simplify the complexity of an occasion to is based or explain. The availability of masses of intellectual models is effective to increase the great of wondering which enables the people to take the proper selection and to address all types of situations. By hacking a person's thoughts, intellectual models make use of the instinct and memory of the individual within a particular and powerful way to get a effective result or to resolve any sort of trouble in ordinary existence. Mental fashions contain of theories which advise internal representation inside the process of thinking.

Mental fashions may be as compared to the diagrams. The motive is that the diagrams assist you to get new ideas whilst you make a scan for them. In a diagram, using a image enables to recognition on an abstract idea. Similarly, in case you make test mental models, you will get the rationale of reasoning concerning abstract standards or ideas. Mental models are awesome and finite and they're not applicable for the illustration of infinite sequences. But they're used for the reason of finite cognitive sources. Anyone can enhance his or her imaginative and prescient with the assist of mental models. It is essential as every person can follow the way of operating inside the international by following an internal photograph provided via the mental models. Mental fashions assist someone to find out a way for the presentation of description related to authentic, hypothetical, remembered or imaginary conditions.

What Cannot Be Described as Mental Models?

There are many proposals furnished by way of cognitive scientists to give an explanation for the way presentation of the mind to describe the arena as an image. Other humans argue that people describe the world thinking about the logical formulas. People, who receive the life of mental fashions, don't take delivery of these arguments. Mental models are not intellectual pix because it doesn't describe a set attitude. Logical formulas can't be defined as mental fashions as they can't produce reasoning through scanning and describe handiest spatial family members. Possibility distributions aren't the equal intellectual models as they describe limitless possibilities simultaneously while every mental version describes a unique possibility. Network representations can not also be described as mental fashions as they cannot produce reasoning and are also dependent based on pre-particular fashions.

History of Mental Models

Mental fashions describe real, imaginary, or hypothetical situations psychologically. In the yr of 1896, Charles Sanders Peirce, an American philosopher, postulated a diagram which he had defined as mental fashions of the world. Later, in the 12 months of 1943, Kenneth Craik, a Scottish psychologist suggested the identical idea. He explained that the human thoughts expects events and describes basics with the aid of building small-scale fashions of the actual world. He additionally thought that the premise of human inference is verbal guidelines. In the year of 1922, Ludwig Wittgenstein, an American philosopher, defined intellectual models much like architect's fashions of constructional work, the complicated molecular shape of biologist's fashions or physicist's diagram to give an explanation for the interaction between the debris of rely.

The ebook "Mental Models" written by way of Phil Johnson-Laird changed into posted in the year of 1983. In this book, he made the argument that the human mind builds intellectual models, consequences of knowledge, notion, reminiscence, imagination, and comprehensive discourse. After that, cognitive scientists had started to research the manner of a baby's questioning process to build a mental model. They additionally started to find out the manner to convey out reasoning, feeling, and mind through mental models.

What Does the Theory of Mental Models Have to Say?

Every mental model describes a opportunity. Its creation correlates to the development of the arena. But it includes symbols for possibility, acceptability, and contradiction and many extra.

Mental models are exemplary insofar as viable which are their segments and relations correlated to those of the situations which they describe. They are based totally on visual pics and also describe abstractions. So, they're wonderful to explain all varieties of conditions.

Mental fashions are effective to explain induction, elimination, and outline. With a legitimate elimination, the inference contains all sorts of fashions of the homes. Within an induction, knowledge reduces fashions of the opportunities and so the inference extends beyond the information provided. Within abduction, expertise brings up new principles to provide an outline.

When there is a demand for several alternative intellectual models, it will become difficult. Generally, human beings make errors once they forget about the possibilities of intellectual models.

Mental models describe best the fact. So, they count on the event of organized and compelling benefits whilst reasoning considers an unfaithful state of affairs. Mental models provide a guideline approximately the ideas which can be feasible comparing to not possible.

The content, as well as expertise inside the intellectual fashions, enables to regulate the meaning of a phrase such as though.

Importance of Mental Models

Mental fashions are a simplified description of the actual-world as customers want for handling occasions or matters. People make use of them to acquire their dreams. People can increase a extensive range of community inclusive of advanced ideas by means of the acquisition of intellectual fashions. By following mental models, you could find out the approaches to build predictions within your environment so long as your interest to looking something might be centered thru a model. When you may accumulate any intellectual version, you may get a description of the framework, idea, or worldwide view. By carrying these descriptions inside your mind, you will be capable of interpret the world and recognize the connection among events and matters. For example, mental fashions of supply as well as demand assist to understand the operating precept of the financial system.

Small-scale mental models have the relation to belief, logic, cognition, and reasoning as they create a fundamental part of conceptual information. Mental fashions are considered for making use of in the future as they assist to increase productivity, creativity, lectures, writing an shrewd publish and keeping smart conversation. They are high-quality to find out the ways to accumulate know-how of the whole thing. Once processing mental fashions within your head, you may regularly enhance an intuitive recognition of the big ideas in the course of many fields. It will increase your understanding skill in addition to mental level while you will collect intellectual models.

By the usage of mental fashions, you can growth your questioning capacity and you could make use of them to any walk of existence. If you can acquire numerous intellectual fashions, your creativity will even enhance on a massive scale. You will collect the strength to study perception into distinctive processes inside the world. Mental fashions make a contribution to spreading out your fashionable tendency that is critical for great expertise and intellectual mastering. If you want to accumulate mental models, you'll have to include your way of wondering and know-how ideas. They will assist you to extract meaningful ideas and records for an occasion or a issue. If you location intellectual models inside your mind, it is going to be advantageous to boost up your learning, thinking, and expertise capability.

Difference Between Mental Models and Real Models

Real models provide an explanation for real events and try to make the right prediction. On the opposite hand, mental models are descriptions of the right predictions considering the state of affairs or occasion.

Real models assume real occasions. Mental models contain the assimilation of intellectual templates for acquiring intuition associated some thing or event.

Real fashions are mounted within hard data. Mental models comprise a wide variety of Content-Free Content which is abstract.

Real fashions involve restrictions which might be accomplished or what are counseled to be accomplished consistent with actual fashions.

Mental fashions encompass interactional performance which includes thinking and belief.

The common customers of the real model are not affordable and are not even all at once much like the models which have applied and used by the software developers. As a end result of this, there may be a gap among the developer's science of reasoning and the belief of users. Mental fashions don't have this form of hole.

You can utilize intellectual models to enhance an instinctive attention of natural in addition to human tactics. There are of limitless mental models existed. If you could gather a touch little bit of those giant things, you may accept many challenges in life. In Physics and engineering, mental fashions are existed to provide an explanation for numerous matters in the complete universe. If you think about the blessings of those intellectual models, for instance, it may be stated that the satisfactory intellectual model permits for locating out new technologies. The development of technology is high quality to build roads and bridges for better communication. Moreover, the improvement of technologies is even beneficial for travelling to outer space.

Applications of intellectual fashions in different regions will decorate your creativity as well as resourceful capacity in distinct fields. You will gain the electricity of expertise of an overview for almost the whole lot by means of applying mental fashions. Mental fashions will help you to be supercharged such as fantastic talents and additionally to be a genius.

Chapter 3: Mental Models For Personal Happiness

You might also have heard the expression, "What you spot is the aspect which you get." It infers that our attitude on the world hinders our ability to stumble upon it. Few might cope with the way that an man or woman who has never experienced love of their lives has a lot of problem locating, retaining up, or assisting a top of the line relationship. Likewise on the off hazard that you've skilled formative years in servile destitution, it takes a variety of individual alternate before you could live with bounty efficiently.

Oozing a quiet, intentional truth is the thriller sauce to flourishing during normal life, do not you concur?

In any case, that allows you to achieve this, we've to attend to an issue. Your internal pundit. The sower of uncertainty, powered by means of damaged molding. Like an stressful spring up, it maintains annoying you with messages that divert you. That pestering little voice. "I can't do it due to [fill in unimportant fact]".

It persuades you to waver… to stop…

You abstain from creating a pass to accomplish your targets, your fantasies or simply to complete stuff whilst all is stated in finished. Your inward pundit persuades you that your snug secure area is simply too comfortable to even keep in mind leaving.

For what motive is it so tough to act with out uncertainty and anxiety? Your thoughts is going for walks a few broken intellectual models. Over our lifetimes, we as an entire receive restricting convictions which can be received via media, youth or unrepresentative reviews.These intellectual models keep us grounded rather than unfastened and certain.

So as to flourish, we have to supplant mistaken contents with the perfect ones. Since whatever you can allow your self recognise, you aren't very old/geeky/fats/moronic or some thing to improve your lifestyles. You are marvelously you and you could have a flourishing lifestyles!

Here are eight instances of intellectual fashions you have to embrace so that it will flourish in this existence.

Acknowledge the world for what it is well worth

For one thing, you need to create articulate acknowledgment of the world you live in.

There are a brilliant deal of awkward certainties in existence that we strive to avoid. Awkward actualities, merciless materials. The international may appear to be unreasonable, but it is truly no longer. The world simply is. There isn't any inalienable goodness or disagreeableness about it. It is only a meeting of things in being.

So end placing your head in the sand—slowly inhale and perceive the reality approximately it. Go up against yourself with the real international. Try now not to gloss over it, yet moreover do not get maneuvered into misrepresented concerns of destiny.

As you renowned how things can be, you can make movements to properly enhance them.

Assume legal responsibility to your lifestyles

You are the essential associate on your lifestyles and, at last, the one especially on the way to consistently mind. You are likewise the one with the maximum instant impact to your life. That implies you are liable for where you turn out to be.

You can also were controlled an lousy hand, however there is no reshuffling the deck. You can simply play the playing cards you have. It's dependent upon you to progress nicely.

In the event that you don't take care of something on your existence, change your disposition towards it or change the condition. Create dynamic adapting methods. Try not to accuse other people, God or the universe. You have unrestrained choice; you're on top of things. Take the treasured view to look toward yourself for development.

three. No self centeredness

Self centeredness is an overwhelming feeling. It's so useless to feel pissed off approximately your self. Regardless of how reasonable, it's miles toxic.

Nothing is picked up through taking element in this decaying attitude. You are down and out? You are plain tremendous? You are 30 and as yet residing in your mother's cellar? Your life may additionally honestly suck, but you cannot stay in self indulgence considering then matters will by no means display signs and symptoms of exchange!

Suck it up. Acknowledge your situation and plan to decorate it. Feeling annoyed about your self just exacerbates things. Lose the injured individual mentality. Learn you may change your self and the situation.

four. Reclassify disappointment in a gaining knowledge of understanding

Disappointment has a chief shame in western lifestyle. When you return up brief, you're a failure. An excessive number of individuals be given that by using one way or another you need to have the choice to win at once. All matters taken into consideration, that won't occur. So why now not provide your self consent to suck and bomb during ordinary lifestyles.

Gain from your slip-ups. You are not a failure seeing that you have got fizzled! The real washouts are the ones that don't try, or who give up too swiftly. The character who falls flat and receives back up is eventually the champ.

Make an attempt no longer to don't forget a to be goal as the meaning of your prosperity. Rather, see gaining ground as development. It may not be a directly line to flawlessness, yet trying to push in advance, thru sadness and mastering is truely fulfillment!

5. Dread is your guide

As you tour via life you will at instances end, incapacitated by dread. Feel the dread and make a move in any case. Except if you are going to win a Darwin grant, you had been maximum possibly destined for success.

Dread offers you where you want to head, however you want to take a bounce. Give dread a threat to reveal some thing you need to do. Push via. Give dread a hazard to be your foreboding manual for flourishing.

6. Consider your passing

Great new each person! We are for the most element going to kick the bucket.

Alright, so perhaps that isn't always such extraordinary news, however it is legitimate. Utilize this as an replace that a while is restricted. One day you may be no greater. It can be the next day; it could be in 80 years. The majority of your little triviality, fears and jealousies ought to fail to measure up to the sizeable difficult to understand nothingness that anticipates you. So why now not take benefit of this awesome lifestyles of yours?

Set apart the attempt to head up towards yourself with this drawing close fate, and cheer which you are as but alive!

Time to comprehend life a whole lot extra with the aid of going for broke and gaining floor towards even the most honest of objectives.

7. Try not to take lifestyles excessively true

What is the importance of lifestyles? What is an extremely good significance? On the off chance which you go down that hare gap, you'll land up with this solution: The significance of life is to live.

It's not extremely grave, but it is fantastically noteworthy. Culture and early life may contend some thing else, however the significance of self-assertive activities, parameters and people is generally misrepresented. There is no vital extra great general to gain, no higher purpose aside from the one you provide your self thru living.

So loosen up. There isn't always a checkpoint you want to head to perform a fulfilling existence. It's simply not excessively real! It is to be delighted in at whatever factor potential. You choose the way you need to stay, so why not relax no matter what people try to assist you to know.

8. Live in the now

To wrap things up, to in reality flourish, you should stay in the now. Figure out how to relinquish your psyche. Quit pursuing misplaced minutes and foreseeing capacity fates.

Your forecasts are for the most component off, and your recollections are remixes of unalterable occasions. Rather, discern out the way to in reality come across what is at once before you, no denying yet greedy the now. Regardless of whether or not it's via sports, nature, or contemplation, grasp the present.

Adjusting these intellectual models may not be a easy task, and it might not occur without any forethought. However, at the off risk that you help yourself to don't forget them and make little strides closer to your targets, you may see after a while that your programming can be changed and it'll amazingly have an effect on your existence.

•ROADMAP TO HAPPINESS: THE MASLOW'S HIERARCHY OF NEEDS

How could we grow to be upbeat? It's inquiry that has been posed on the grounds that the start of time and spoke back by way of thinkers, masters, and – all the extra as of past due – clinicians. One of them changed into Abraham Maslow. He detailed 'Maslow's Hierarchy of Needs', otherwise called the 'pyramid of joy.' It made up his 1943 paper A Theory of Human Motivation and was distributed in Psychological Review.

All in all, what exactly is Maslow's Hierarchy of Needs and the way would possibly we benefit from this pyramid model at the off hazard that we need to be cheerful?

Maslow's Hierarchy of Needs is an inspirational hypothesis in mind technology comprising of a 5-level model of human desires, frequently appeared as various leveled tiers inner a pyramid. Maslow's pyramid is separated into five levels of necessities, from the bottom of the chain of importance upwards:

- physiological

- protection

- love and having a place

- esteem

- self-actualisation

Maslow's Hierarchy of Needs: the five stages

Physiological desires

These are organic and physical requirements, inclusive of respiration, nourishment, water, and relaxation. At the factor while these necessities are not happy, they become the principle aspect we're distracted with.

Security desires

These are matters, as an example, physical protection, and requirements for domestic, paintings, pay, and well-being. Without satisfaction of those requirements, an person continuously feels unsure and unprotected.

three. Love and having a place wishes

These arrangement with our desires for profound relational institutions, top notch own family connections, companionships, and sexual closeness. Without them, we can also land up discouraged or revel in forlornness.

Regard needs

These are necessities which includes self belief, fact, accomplishment, and being seemed by way of others.

five. Self-cognizance needs

These arrangement with inventiveness, suddenness and critical thinking. They are met on the off chance that we are able to progress towards becoming all that we are ready for buying to be. Self-finishing people have a grounded feeling of prosperity and fulfillment. What's greater, a feeling of stunningness, surprise, and appreciation about existence.

Maslow noticed that his chain of significance is a general portrayal. And keeping in mind that he at the start expressed that humans need to fulfill lower stage wishes earlier than advancing directly to greater massive stage development desires, he later explained that fulfillment of requirements isn't an "all-or-none" surprise. Accordingly, degrees aren't constant, and every need does not need to be satisfied a hundred percent to have the choice to move to more sizeable levels.

Maslow's Hierarchy of Needs: insufficiency needs

Things being what they're, taking a gander at this chain of importance, how could we turn out to be satisfied? Maslow referred to as the decrease four stages 'insufficiency desires' (D-wishes): at the off danger that they 're no longer met, it impacts our mental health and hinders our inclination for improvement, self-rule, persona, and greatness. The final, pinnacle level is the alleged 'improvement' or 'being desires' (B-needs).

Much of the time, lack needs emerge due to difficulty. At the factor when they're overlooked, they may be said to propel individuals greater. To be sure, notion to fulfill these requirements finally ends up greater grounded the greater they may be denied. For instance, the extra drawn out an man or woman abandons nourishment, the hungrier they may turn into.

Pyramid of joy: 'Development' or 'Being' needs

Maslow's 'development' or 'being' needs don't clearly originate from a lack of something, yet as a substitute from a craving to expand as an person. When those improvement needs have been pretty lots fulfilled, one may be notion to arrive at the highest point of the pyramid of joy – the maximum multiplied stage, called 'self-awareness'.

When any individual has met their lack wishes, the concentration to self-cognizance starts and we – irrespective of whether or not simply at an intuitive stage — start to don't forget further mind concerning our truth, purpose and importance for the duration of everyday lifestyles.

Every one of us can likely climb the chain of command closer to a diploma of self-attention. In any case, development is frequently disillusioned by means of an incapability to fulfill lower stage wishes. Obviously, beneficial encounters, as an instance, misplaced employment, depression or uneasiness, medical troubles, and many may make humans vacillate among ranges of the delight chain of command. To make sure, no longer all os will climb the progressive machine in one manner for ever: we may additionally move back and forth between the special want kinds.

Maslow's Pyramid: improvement of the Hierarchy of Needs

It's vital to take note of that later, in the course of the Nineteen Sixties and 70s, Maslow delivered exceptional tiers to the pinnacle part of the necessities pyramid, which include 'psychological', 'fashionable' and, after 'self finishing touch', 'superb quality' wishes. He tested what keeps self-actualising individuals — those at the best point of the joy pyramid — roused. He located that these people look for such things as reality, goodness, class, greatness, and so forth.

Psychological wishes

These contain facts and getting, hobby, investigation, requirement for importance and consistency.

Stylish desires

The gratefulness and quest for elegance, stability, shape, and so on.

eight. Amazing excellent desires

A human is spurred with the aid of values which rise above beyond the sense of self and man or woman self (e.G., encounters with nature, appeal, tasteful and sexual encounters, self assurance, selflessness, the intensity of graciousness, and so forth.)

Rather than being pursuits that consist of private situation, these characteristics rise above the man or woman. By together with these need types into Maslow's Hierarchy of Needs the clinician addressed analysis approximately the nonappearance of wants to know, needs for class, and needs for fact, in his particular version of the pyramid of joy.

•CHANGE YOUR THINKING CHANGE YOUR LIFE

They nation an inspirational mentality decides how some distance we go at some point of regular lifestyles, and everything else among. In any case, does this follow when you're in a state of affairs where you experience undervalued, segregated, and misjudged?

Our frame of thoughts impacts our connections, bliss, way of lifestyles, and fulfillment. Building up an inspirational demeanor makes a massive difference however our situations. Factually a large part of the people conceived are hopeful normally, and the alternative half are cynical. Which manner there's a half opportunity that you see existence thru a negative focal point.

Indeed, even the hopeful man or woman will assume that its hard every so often to have an inspirational body of thoughts due from lifestyles encounters, effect, and social molding. So whichever you are,,,, Today is every other day for clean begins. Disregard the whole lot your mentality has manufactured from your lifestyles, and begin once more. Adjust it. Sand the harsh spots, and start constructing up an inspirational outlook that changes you into the man or woman you want to be. Here are a few exclusive approaches how, and where to start.

Building up an inspirational frame of mind

Building up an inspirational body of mind should be our pinnacle need for any fulfillment. First we've to investigate what an inspirational body of mind resembles, and the way certain portions of our character reflect it. We likewise want to perceive any cause why individuals see us with a specific intention in thoughts.

Recollect that others can not guess what you is probably questioning, so they measure you through social standing, non-verbal communique, and correspondence. In the event that you discover a larger part of people brushing off you, disliking you perhaps your frame of thoughts is distorting what your identification is. The manner in which you see your self displays again to you from other people.

For what cause is that this big? Since how we perceive with others makes a decision our prosperity, or disappointment in all that we do.

Your frame of mind is an articulation to the outside universe of what your identity is. It would not make a distinction if you're correct or wrong. What makes a difference is that you increase an inspirational mentality that pals with people such that gives you what you want.

Initially this may appear control, but as a wellknown rule it's called courting constructing talents. Furthermore, with out them we won't get plenty of anywhere. Here are a few different ways to accumulate an inspirational body of mind.

Shape your disposition with appreciation: Without appreciation we end up disheartened, unpleasant, and angry. Bend over backward to understand a soul of appreciation in each situation. Look for the most unimportant matters to acclaim, and you'll discover grand things begin to occur surrounding you.

It's some thing but difficult to have an inspirational body of mind whilst the whole thing's ideal, except shouldn't some thing be said about when it's clearly not? You can not ascend a high mountain on a easy surface.. You need profound cleft to assist your following level. The profound fissure are scars – tough problems which have made you extra grounded, and more potent. At the factor while regarded with difficulties our actual man or woman consistently seems. On the off danger that you could hold close an uplifting mentality at some point of the crucial point in time your achievements will come to be relentless.

Win Big: We all realise the sector is loaded up with champs, and screw ups, however what isolates the two? Clearly diligent work by myself does not guarantee fulfillment. The setting apart line is a wonderful perspective paying little mind to situations. This is the issue that isolates champs from disasters at some stage in life. Exceptionally effective individuals building up a triumphant body of thoughts that ultimately makes effective effects.

Remain positive The excellent method to exchange situations is to trade our body of mind towards them. We have to grasp an inspirational body of mind, and expect total liability for every condition we land up in. We should discover answers for tough difficulties even as evacuating physiological obstructions that effect most capacity.

This will alternate any point of view, and make existence a superior spot to stay. There are constantly things to grouse approximately, yet how they're handled has a enormous impact. There are solutions to every condition we are facing when they may be visible through an inspirational frame of mind.

Chapter 4: Mental Models For Making Decisions

Making decisions may be very hard. While a few people are clearly decisive, others battle with choices on a every day foundation, although the stakes aren't really that excessive. Simply having alternatives is overwhelming, and the notion of creating the wrong selection is haunting. At a few factor, everybody - even people who can generally make a preference in a second - will struggle with a choice, whether it's at paintings or in their non-public lives. Mental fashions can help each person with you make a decision at any given time. In this chapter, we'll discover the maximum beneficial fashions for choice-making and a few tangible methods on how to appoint them.

#1: Inversion

One of the most well-known intellectual fashions, inversion is the method of wondering backwards. It comes from the phrase "invert," this means that to turn upside down. If you're suffering with you decide, it may assist to have a look at what you don't need to appear first, after which paintings backwards. Charlie Munger says, "A lot of success in existence and enterprise comes from understanding what you want to keep away from: early death, a awful marriage, etc." Rather than trying to wrack your mind about what you wish will manifest and the way to get there, recollect rather what you don't need to appear.

As an example, permit's say you're looking to make a selection about what rental to hire. You have a handful which you truly like, and aren't certain which to select. Rather than looking at all the things and amenities the special residences must provide, use the inversion mental model and reflect onconsideration on what you don't like or need. Instead of considering what would make an condominium the precise domestic, consider what might make an apartment awful. You become with this listing:

Hand-washing dishes each night time

Not being capable of do laundry whenever I need

Not having the gap to have a celebration

Needing to drive over 1/2 an hour to work

With a picture of the worst rental to your mind, you could identify the specific stuff you don't need. Now, while looking at apartments, you are capable of do away with lots of them.

Inversion is also a completely beneficial mental model to use while thinking about investments and shares. Think about what could should show up as a way to realize you've made a awful funding. You'll be able to discern out what level of danger you're inclined to tackle and make a selection consequently. Inversion can shield you from large regrets, like dropping lots of cash, as it forces you to don't forget worse-case eventualities. It's additionally a amazing approach for solving troubles.

#2: Second-order wondering

When you're seeking to make a choice, you reflect onconsideration on the possible outcomes of your selections. As an example, let's say you're trying to make a choice approximately a work challenge, and which part of it to awareness on first. You're very comfortable with one aspect of it, however the different element is intimidating. First-order questioning is what you're doing when you just skim the surface of your decision. You assume, "If I paintings on the component I'm familiar with first, I can reach the primary closing date benchmark faster." Second-order questioning, but, requires you to observe the effects of the outcomes. This is an crucial intellectual version as it reveals issues that remain hidden with first-order questioning.

Let's employ 2nd-order wondering on this paintings challenge example. Yes, first-order questioning tells you that you'll reach the first cut-off date quicker if you attention on the component you're acquainted with first, but the impact of that is which you are then left with a more intimidating component on your very last deadline. You will cope with an multiplied degree of stress, and mixed with your loss of consolation with the mission, you would possibly paintings an awful lot slower. Because you used second-order questioning in this situation, you decide to tackle the harder components of the task first, leaving the simpler work - which isn't as traumatic - for your final closing date.

Second-order wondering is a chunk like playing a chess sport together with your choices. You appearance beforehand and recall what would possibly manifest based at the alternatives you make now, after which consider what else should happen. Second-order questioning prevents you from making short choices and dealing with unforeseen results, a lot of which could convey up even harder choices. There's less surprise and stress on your life while you use this mental model.

#three: Pareto Efficiency

Sometimes, you may't improve some thing with out sacrificing first-class somewhere else. That idea is known as the Pareto Efficiency. This mental model is traditionally based on economics and springs from Vilfredo Pareto, an Italian engineer and economist. Pareto's Efficiency pops up if you have to make your mind up on a way to use restrained resources most correctly, and you may't make each person glad. In economics, this takes place while you may't improve one group or individual's lifestyles better with out making every other group's worse. In engineering, it's about sacrificing exceptional in one area of a product or task for the sake of another area.

The purpose of the Pareto Efficiency mental model isn't equity; it's really figuring out what the maximum efficient distribution is. That means there are a number of areas in lifestyles wherein it likely shouldn't be used, however in a work placing, it may be very beneficial for tough choice-making. It also can be beneficial for personal budgeting, due to the fact you handiest have a lot money at your disposal. You can't circulate $100 into your meals finances without taking that cash from some different class.

The useful aspect approximately this intellectual model is it strips away dreams approximately trying extra resources and what you could do with them. Instead, you're forced to focus on what you have got in the front of you. Reality might be cruel, but it's all we've got. The Pareto Efficiency allow you to prioritize and simply think about the best, maximum productive desire.

#four: Crowdsourcing

This mental version is based on the idea that asking a huge institution of humans what they think can help a person or business enterprise make a selection. It's very useful in case you've narrowed down your choices to a handful or even simply two alternatives, and aren't sure what the very last choice must be. Crowdsourcing has been around a long term in the form of surveys, and now, inside the age of the internet, it's very easy to get a big range of opinions.

Crowdsourcing is a awesome tool for selections about merchandise, because it we could the inventor or business enterprise parent out what human beings will sincerely like. Rather than sit around looking to bet what customers need, you could simply provide them with options and ask, "Which do you want first-rate?" The idea may be broadened even more, so customers are given loose reign to decide on some thing. Hasbro used net balloting to choose their new Monopoly pieces, whilst Anheuser-Busch once evolved a new craft beer with brewmasters, clients, and others.

The Crowdsourcing mental version believes within the "understanding of the group," and that through gathering as many solutions as possible, it's less complicated to discover the proper one. This belief doesn't always maintain up, but that doesn't mean it shouldn't be at least taken into consideration when constructing a latticework of mental fashions.

#5. The Eisenhower Matrix

How do you decide what's vital at paintings and in lifestyles? What have to an enterprise's or an man or woman's priorities be? The Eisenhower Matrix (additionally known as the Eisenhower Box) offers a first rate shape for figuring these items out. It's based on how President Eisenhower prepared his existence and optimized his time management and productivity. It's simple, so it's useful for pretty much everyone.

The idea is which you separate your actions based on four quadrants: urgent and important; crucial, however no longer pressing; urgent, but no longer important; and neither urgent nor important. The first quadrant is for obligations which you want to do first due to the fact in case you don't do them, there's a terrible effect. As an instance, you've got a undertaking due in an hour, and also you aren't done yet. If you don't finish it, you'll be in problem. The challenge wishes to be completed before you do whatever else.

Quadrant 2 consists of tasks which are important, but no longer time-sensitive. These are lengthy-term goals that line up with your values, like getting a college degree, reading extra books about your dream profession, and saving for retirement. These are responsibilities that get done in increments and thru regular commitment. Quadrant 3 is for duties which can be time-sensitive or urgent, so they appear vital, but that may not truely be the case. If your career or non-public existence doesn't suffer because of waiting or delegating the project to someone else, they belong in Quadrant three.

The last Quadrant is for responsibilities that don't achieve something. They don't advantage your personal or expert existence, or contribute on your lengthy-term desires. Most people spend plenty of time simply striking out, looking at our phones, scrolling via Facebook or Instagram, and looking TV we don't virtually like. It might be not possible to eliminate this segment completely because all of us want to region out every so often, however you should spend the least quantity of your time in Quadrant 4. Organizing your life and duties with the Eisenhower Matrix mental model allows making a decision what definitely topics.

#6: Probabilistic Thinking

While used frequently in math and technological know-how, Probabilistic Thinking can be hired in different regions of existence, as properly. Its basic cause is to estimate the chance of positive results the use of essential statistics. Decisions can be hard to make because there's such a lot of elements at play and a lot records. If you're trying to pick from numerous options, the Probabilistic Thinking version can help. It enables you realistically observe the likelihood of all the results generated by way of any selection.

As an example, allow's say you are trying to decide what jobs to use for. You have pretty a long listing, however don't want to use to they all because of how a good deal time on the way to take. You need to spend your time and power at the programs which you really have a real shot at nailing. To use Probabilistic Thinking, you will studies the roles and businesses, paying special interest to the qualifications they're searching out, the varieties of people the enterprise currently has on team of workers, your experience and qualifications, and so on.

With the statistics you've gathered, you can begin Probabilistic Thinking. You decide you're much more likely to get an interview for a activity that prefers at the least three years of experience (you've got 4) than a job that prefers 7 years. You additionally see that the various businesses have personnel that graduated out of your alma mater and cost volunteer work, which you frequently are trying to find out. Using Probabilistic Thinking and getting a strong sense of odds, you may reduce your wide variety of alternatives and make more particular selections. This intellectual version can also be used for problem-fixing and figuring out the chance of answers becoming fact.

#7: Paradox of Choice

This mental model is named after a 2004 ebook by using psychologist Barry Schwartz. In his e-book The Paradox of Choice: Why Less Is More, Schwartz laid out his thesis that having too many options makes it tougher to come to a decision. He became particularly speaking about clients and shopping tension, however this idea may be carried out to different areas of life. Like other mental models on this phase on choice-making, the Paradox of Choice values simplicity over complexity. To avoid being paralyzed via a plethora of alternatives, a person wishes to simplify and reduce their alternatives to make the pleasant selection.

As an example, allow's say you are attempting to determine what sort of TV to buy. You begin through compiling a listing of all the TVs in your rate variety, but comprehend that there are in order that many alternatives, you can research for all time and never honestly make a choice. Paradox of Choice informs you the nice course of motion is to pause. You can narrow your selections by means of adding extra perimeters similarly to fee range, like size, display decision, and number of ports.

In the years since the book, many have puzzled the validity that "much less is more," at least in certain situations. Schwartz himself stated the key's locating the sweet spot between providing variety, which is ideal, and supplying so much that the options are paralyzing. The Paradox of Choice still remains a good intellectual version to bear in mind while going through decisions. The "less is extra" philosophy and procedure of figuring out what without a doubt subjects also can help whilst you're trying to assume more simply.

#eight: Reversible vs. Irreversible

When you're going through a handful of decision alternatives at once, the Reversible vs. Irreversible mental model may be very beneficial. You divide up the choices into classes: one that may be reversed and ones that cannot. Looking at choices in this mild can help you make a decision how a good deal danger you want to tackle in the interim, and what kind of time you want to put into making this choice. You can also use this version whilst you're thinking about one decision genuinely through asking, "Can this be reversed? If it is able to't, am I ok with that?"

What are some examples of this mental version in movement? Again, let's say you're purchasing for a TV and are leaning toward one specially. You haven't pulled the cause however, due to the fact you're concerned about making the wrong preference. When you operate the Reversible vs. Irreversible mental version, you comprehend that you may constantly return the TV in case you don't love it. You don't want to spend numerous time agonizing over a reversible choice. On the opposite hand, quitting your task is an irreversible selection. You have to sincerely reflect onconsideration on this choice on a deeper degree because you may't just come returned in your boss and ask for your task returned if making a decision you made the incorrect desire.

The Reversible vs. Irreversible intellectual model can prevent a number of time in case you cope with decision-making all day. While it isn't an excuse to act rashly or without any thought, it does assist you prioritize which choices you must invest your energy in. This intellectual model is likewise helpful while hassle-fixing and looking to determine which solutions to attempt out. If a risky answer is reversible, you'll be a lot greater comfortable picking it over a solution this is each volatile and irreversible.

Chapter 5: Eye-Opening Problem-Solving

It is a not unusual phenomenon of human beings looking to remedy the daily issues completely with their minds. However, the solutions to the problems that gift to an man or woman's existence regularly have a deep root as the answer. The most advised method to go about existence issues is locating a step forward in mind and styles of living. It is a hard venture for those elements of change to come back approximately with the aid of looking at them as a short-term form of technique.

Successful people have the tendency of reweaving the issues they stumble upon with a view of a long time angle. The befit of this type of metallic placing is it makes it smooth to arrive at answers. These answers regularly have the potential of creating an man or woman be happy in his or her existence. A accurate depiction is a person who is trying to find a process together with his or her aim to improve his or her happiness. However, there is a positive purpose that would be unfavorable to an character if he or she uses it as the cause to discover a job. The cause is pursuing a activity to satisfy what is socially right and now not what his or her pursuits are.

The different depiction might be that of a figure who's aiming to settle his or her daughter. The primary intention of this act is to make his or her lady settle. However, there are cases where it's miles a disaster for a female who needs independence. The reason is the act has the capability of causing her extra troubles while she is married. This makes her parents find themselves in a state of affairs that is helpless than in which they had been before. These depictions prove the element that the answers to a trouble are supposed so that you can increase and man or woman happiness. The solution is also supposed to pass a notch higher to enhancing an character's soul empowerment and ascension to a degree that is peaceful for their lifestyles.

There is a certain analogy that is used to explain the technique of fixing problems the use of the third eye. The analogy is using objectiveness like God to resolve his or her problems. One is supposed so that it will open his or her 1/3 eye because it creates a good connection to other geographical regions of fixing troubles. It may sound overwhelming, however the two physical eyes are simplest tasked with the function of seeing the physicality of the sector. The 1/3 eye is tasked with the function of seeing the facts this is non-physical. This consists of distinctive interpretations of lifestyles happenings. One can describe the 1/3 eye-beginning as the middle of instinct. Opening this eye calls for numerous matters, which includes:

Peer Review Your Perspectives

The everyday lifestyles of a person has not anything that is right or wrong in regards to uncommon circumstances positioned apart. Right and incorrect tend to be relative terms with regards to the aspect an character wants to pass. The not unusual school of concept is that achievement is doing what one loves until the give up of lifestyles. These are most important locations an individual has to reach. However, there may be an element that several people generally tend to miss it. The detail is that the two terms of proper and incorrect are what's used to method the journey for an individual to be successful.

One is discouraged from questioning the 2 words are the vacation spot for the adventure of being a hit. A individual is called a success in the occasion that he or she is strolling a adventure that he or she is usually getting to know and developing from it. Successful people do what they love in the occasion that they see each second that offers itself to them as an possibility. There are billions of human beings which might be in lifestyles currently. This makes the view of the possibility to be distinct among them. Therefore, it's far essential for an man or woman in order to locate his form of possibility.

The millennial we are presently living is packed with peers who are annoyed almost every day. The purpose of frustration is the notion of the whole lot seeming to seem like being everlasting. You aren't presupposed to wine about the cubicle form of task you have and having the quit concept of sticking there. This is unfavorable because it diminishes your desire to be successful. It could be very important for any person who is looking for to achieve success in being able to recognize that there are training in the journey of lifestyles. It is also crucial to include those instructions. Embracing mistakes makes someone be capable of attain absolutely the nation of being a hit. The sense at the back of it is that a person could be developing resultseasily to turning into a higher version of himself or herself.

There is a first-rate purpose why numerous humans tend to suffer on the subject of a overview of thoughts. It is due to the duty aspect this is worried in them. Accountability includes an person searching at the reflection of his or her mind. The system is crucial because it has the capacity of shifting blames on one-of-a-kind problems of lifestyles to possession. You are meant which will see opportunities from the hassle that life provides and an character from this manner. It is a idea that may be used across all of the angles of lifestyles from social, educational to paintings-lifestyles of an individual.

You are purported to capable of have a leaser attention on the classes from a lifestyles occasion. This brings the school of idea that an character isn't always presupposed to reflect onconsideration on the hassle. Try no longer responsible people around you as the cause of the problems which you enjoy in your every day lifestyles. Every scenario that life has the ability of fixing an person has the capability of being a turnaround. These classes are frequently located anywhere, and it is someone's mission on the way to spot them. They have the ability of making an character develop. When it turns into a difficult challenge to find the instructions on this technique, an man or woman may be able to ask folks who are round him or her via asking them questions on what he or she will improve in his or her existence. The main intention is usually for you to exchange your attitude.

Find Your Own Flaws

There are sure varieties of thinking that fill the regular world of an person. You are subjected to suppose of getting a a success enterprise or a typically a hit lifestyles. There are other elements that dominate the delusion world of an man or woman. These different elements are winning the lottery each day, having an amazing form of hair, and a super tummy this is flat.

However, there's a less than perfect global which you are supposed so that it will deal with as an person. The reality that we are facing every day is that we are handiest correct at sure things. There are different things which you cause them to satisfactory and some things which can be downright awful regardless of being critical. It can be very hard to address the genuine reality that you can be capable of cope with the whole lot flawlessly. Or on different phrases, it's miles impossible to be an excellent human. The commonplace idea is that of someone who is the head of an organization. This person is vulnerable to having the concept of he or she is the only man or woman who could make an business enterprise to be achieving its goals and goals optimally. This concept is improper if you are such type of character because no one is ideal, nor is any person.

It is essential with a view to locate your flaws because no one is best. The technique of being a success is going a notch higher to turning them into styles of strengths. There are numerous steps you can comply with for you with the intention to achieve success in turning those weaknesses into numerous types of energy.

Recognition of the Weaknesses

It is a tough assignment of turning weaknesses into strength inside the occasion that you deny them. Therefore, the primary task is accepting that you have flaws and locating a way of recognizing them. There are numerous methods to identify these styles of weaknesses, and the maximum common one is taking a character take a look at. It is a complex and tricky method with regards to navigating through it. It is one of the maximum validated strategies across the globe. The process has the tendency to test and organization human beings into 5 popular personalities. The system is focused on five key regions of your personality. They stated character regions consisting of neuroticism, agreeableness, extroversion, attention, and openness.

Get Guidance

It is vital usually to have a consistent notion that not absolutely everyone may be trusted. Opening up about your weakness is a delicate difficulty, and you're required to have someone you have a near dating with. The individual who you are to open up approximately those issues must be shiny and wise. This will come up with a higher insight into a way to deal with this type of problem. Such people can act as mentors considering the fact that they give you guidance to obtain your goals in life, which might be a measure of fulfillment. These humans may be pals, circle of relatives members, or colleagues you have interaction with at a non-public stage.

three. Being Prepared

There are moments where you can be able to fight weakness you possess in an clean way. The green and smooth approach entails getting first rate styles of guidance. A precise depiction could be that of someone who has a hassle of having misplaced moments he or she travels by himself or herself. Such a person can conquer the weak spot of forgetting course through ensuring he or she has a map any moment she or he is travelling. This entails the use of paper maps or GPS packages on either his or her car, tablet, or cellphone. The identical case may be utilized by you when you are at work or at faculty. This involves seeking out greater statistics about the state of affairs you are approximately to deal with or the person that could be involved in it.

Hire the Skills You Lack

Successful is known for acknowledging that they are no best at the entirety they do. This makes them have a low likely hood of handling things that they do no longer recognize. Therefore, the rich are recognised for going the more mile of hiring human beings to fulfill the tasks that they are now not precise at executing them. The technique is fantastic because despite compensating someone's weakness, it offers him with new ideas that he or she will be able to use to better him or herself. You are intended for you to delegate several obligations of your existence to other human beings round you. The duties might be performed correctly within the event that an individual is going a notch higher to empowering those those who are round him or her so as to carry out those responsibilities comfortably.

five. Getting Just Good Enough

At this point, you are capable of understand which you aren't precise at all of the tasks you perform. However, there are other duties that may be found out on a day by day foundation. They can be incorporated with the tasks you understand. The subsequent step would be you going a notch excessive to make sure that you higher your self in both the new capabilities. And the other nice attributes that you use to own. The procedure of getting to be good enough will assist you get thru sure troubles in lifestyles that appear to be very hard. Take an instance of an entrepreneur the usage of popular expertise of entrepreneurship ideas to get thru conditions where generation has failed, along with marketplace evaluation. The process is fine as it makes someone be able to have a clever technique in the entirety he or she does in his or her life.

Looking for a Way to Serve Other People With the Same Problem

There is a common announcement that has an ideology of invention being born from aggravation. This method that for you a good way to gain certain competencies on your life, you need calamities to strike first. It is a hidden form of converting weaknesses into strength. Taking a examine the wealthy humans who've numerous paperwork, improvements will make you have an exciting discovery. The interesting discovery would be that these humans made their fortune from the purpose of helping society. This is irrespective of product or service that they delivered inside the marketplace. Having a eager examine your weaknesses can serve as an opportunity because it has the capacity of main you to a a hit assignment.

Separate Correlation From Causation

Causation and correlation can appear to appear like comparable terms with a blurry line. However, spotting the difference among the two may be very vital for you. This is because it will assist you to interrupt down your efforts on elements in lifestyles that have low price. The method is critical due to the fact nearly the complete international is focused on concentrating on elements that have a high cost. It can take any shape including capabilities, product, and carrier or a character trait.

The truth is that that correlation and causation have the chance of being in life on the same time. However, from the above statistics, causation does now not mean correlation. It is crucial for someone to know the distinction among the 2 terms. Causation may be described because the resulting movement from action has been carried out. For instance, movement A leading to action B. On the opposite hand, correlation may be defined because the resulting relationship among moves. A depiction will be the dating of action A to B. These actions or activities aren't subjected to be the purpose of the opposite while finding their correlation.

There is a positive reason that explains why humans have a difficult venture of differentiating the 2 aspects of thinking. The primary reason is that the human thoughts is constant to finding numerous styles in lifestyles, even inside the occasion that they do now not exist. You are at risk of fabricating certain styles within the event that two variables seem to have a near affiliation. The near association formed with the aid of the thoughts makes these life happenings to appear like they are dependent on each different. It is the cause why people are inclined and brief to implying the motive and impact relationship. This is within the occasion that there may be a established resulting in an independent occasion however.

This act has a unfavorable effect on individual fulfillment. The most important reason is that it is able to lead you to a path of misguided end when you are executing duties together with thing evaluation. Correlation is a statistic tool with regards to thing evaluation. The technique is tasked with the position of depicting the level of relatedness between variables. It is regular to discover that variables do not have a similar reason or impact; this is no matter the variables having a close relationship.

It brings to limelight another description that may be used to consult causation. The description is causation is the connection that exists between the impact and motive of positive movements. There are numerous depictions that may be used to illustrate this phenomenon. They include a person claiming that the procedure of him or her strolling thru the door become the motive he or she broke his or her nostril. The other possibly purpose might be she or he become texting or the use of his or her phone whilst on foot. Therefore, in this context, texting and the occasion of the nose breaking will be the motive why the man or woman broke her or his nose.

There are other phenomena that manifest each and each day that you could have the ability to relate. Take the instance of searching at the purpose of injuries. Performing a issue analysis calls for you to have several issues. They might encompass purple motors, better velocity limits, inclement climate, and young drivers. You can be subjected by using the thoughts to thinks that red motors have the tendency of causing injuries, which isn't the case. Taking a observe younger drivers sparks using facts that claim younger drivers have the ability of inflicting injuries. However, this is not the direct hyperlink of all the road carnages that are skilled. The factors prove it tough to categorize them as causation or correlation.

You can take a deep have a look at the climate and try and classify it as either causation or correlation. Rain will have the potential of making a younger driver cause an twist of fate due to negative visibility. However, it isn't always the direct motive of all of the injuries which can be skilled. Rain could make roads to be slippery and deliver a driving force a tough venture to break, but it isn't always the pressure behind making two cars to collide. Taking a study high velocity has the ability of creating someone purpose an coincidence, and it's far risky. However, the issue for the accident occurring would be malfunctioning of the breaks that are a right away result in injuries.

The procedure of knowledge causation and correlation is a mastered art with the aid of a hit humans. It is a useful way of searching at daily life issues that present an individual. The advantage is it allows someone to avoid making incorrect assumptions based on the information one has. You can be capable to steer people around you, inclusive of your self, with the aid of looking through the vital lenses supplied by this evaluation. It may be a difficult task of you searching at numerous life happenings entirely at the correlating factors. It will become very difficult to discover several answers to certain issues. Therefore, attaining fulfillment for your life requires you to use data because the figuring out issue of the motive with the intention to awareness on the best effect success can convey.

Chapter 6: How To See More Clearly

Have you ever thought of the unique use of binoculars for your life? Binoculars provide us consciousness on things which can be some distance and which can be foreign to us. You can watch as a chook construct a nest and feed its infants, you could watch as a lion hunts its prey, or you can watch the alignment of our sun device. All these uses and lots of more, however, alas, a binocular blinds us from the things which are below our noses. When you pick to apply binoculars, you may best have the a ways view and miss the finer information underneath your nose. To binoculars, it is not possible to see each methods, but in lifestyles, it may be tough however now not not possible. You need to teach your brain to prevent jumping to conclusions and filling inside the blank areas. You can be attentive, but it isn't viable to rely upon what you listen or see to make a full photograph of what is on the floor. It turns into hard due to the fact you might depend upon information from a biased man or woman, or your beliefs and biases may lead you to make a defective judgment. Our built in wires do now not permit us to peer or assume objectively, and it becomes simpler to save you it while we well known that.

This chapter allows you to view the sector as what it's miles, something that most of us conflict with. The mental models on this chapter will assist you to look through false realities and distractions of our lives and allow you to get to the fact as close as you may. They are tools that will assist you extra than you can consider. For instance, we've all heard of the announcing that to make an informed decision on a place that you may not discover to, it would be essential in case you visited it all the four seasons. You can also go to the location in the two worst seasons earlier than making an informed decision. If you go to the vicinity for some days, it'd be unwise to come to a decision basing on that. All gadgets or situations are concern to alternate because of exceptional conditions and occasions. When it involves collecting statistics, there may be no shortcut. You need to get as much data as feasible earlier than making a decision. The manner is probably tedious and overwhelming but very important for higher know-how and intelligence series. Having this mindset encourages you to quite a few facts on any state of affairs or subject matter from special environments, backgrounds, and situations as you can. When you have lots of records at your disposal, you avoid making blind assumptions, inaccurate projections, and snap judgments. To have a broader evaluation of all conditions, allow us to look at specific templates of intellectual models.

Ignore "Black Swans"

This model lets you apprehend the way you must now not permit your questioning to be inspired by means of outliers. Did you realize that Europe at huge believed that the swan was best in white up till the 18th century? They reasoned that they've by no means seen a swan of every other color, and with that absence, they had no cause to trust that there has been a swan of any other coloration. In 1697, it marked the beginning of changing that belief. Willem De Vlamingh, a Dutch explorer, traveled to

Australia. During his exploration, he strolled along the Swan River, and together along with his crew, they saw what turned into new to any European's eyes. They noticed masses of black swans swimming in the river. This new sight made a robust effect, and they rewrote a few tenets in Zoology at the notion that all swans had been white. Imagine if swans have been as many in colors as the colors on the rainbow.

Statistician Nassim Nicholas used the above records to come up with the black swan principle. He takes the black swan as the unpredictable occasions in our lives that purpose fantastic trade in our information and perceptions. Yet, to Nassim, the black swan ought to no longer trade our perceptions or ideals because it is a odd outliner. The black swan need to create attention, however it need to no longer be accounted for every day. Seeing every other coloration of the swan have to were translated that black swans exist in both black and white coloration but have to now not result in throwing out the whole perception system of zoology. For instance, in case you study that a tree became struck through lightning to your neighborhood, you may get nervous, and you can take a similarly step to put in a few lightning rods. Now, must that equal event change your lifestyle? Should you live indoors during after that to avoid being struck by means of lightning? Does it suggest that you must trade towns to keep away from lightning, or should you pass underground and start living like a mole?

According to Taleb, the thinkers earlier than him only took care of the improbabilities. He explained that the surprising might be foretold by way of getting statistics from statistics calculated at the past observations. Taleb stated that the same old happenings did not problem him, however if you need to recognize a state of affairs, you should have a look at it from the extraordinary factor of view. Is it possible to have an know-how of health without a understanding of epidemics? Well, regular is beside the point, and in case you study your social life, you may observe the jumps and shocks in it, however in reality, all we realize about it's far ordinary. It happens because the bell curve does not take note of the large deviations, but on the same time, it makes us think that it has protected all the uncertainties.

Look for Equilibrium Points

There are so many ways we will explain them equilibrium factors mental version, however the easiest is the Boombustology, wherein a small ball lies on a curved form, as proven beneath.

equilibrium

In the 2 diagrams below, equilibrium can simplest be finished if we go away them on my own and allow the ball to find its region. In disequilibrium, the ball does not discover a place to settle. Newton makes use of three laws to explain this model. He used planets to illustrate how gravity behaves among two gadgets. He defined that the sun's gravity is offset through the planet's pace, therefore, equating the powers and developing equilibrium. What is the equilibrium? It is the stability between opposing forces. There unique types of equilibrium. Static equilibrium is whilst the gadget is resting whilst dynamic equilibrium is where there may be a presence of two or extra forces, and that they have equal powers.

Hagstrom Robert suggests us the difference among those two equilibriums inside the Last Liberal Arts. He explains that when a scale has equal weights on both aspects, it represents static equilibrium while our our bodies represent dynamic equilibrium; when our our bodies lose heat to hold the stability with the sugar consumptions

Supply and Demand + Equilibrium

Warren Buffet purchased 11.2 million oz of silver thru Berkshire Hathaway in 1997. In his quit of the 12 months letter, he stated that the inventory had reduced materially, and they had determined collectively with Charlie Munger to boom the charge to equate the forces of deliver and call for. In Boombustology, Mansharamani explains that the most method towards equilibrium is the belief that extended expenses produce new deliver that reduces the fees. It is likewise believed that reduced expenses bring about new call for that, in turn, hikes the costs.

Forces of supply and demand allow us to make knowledgeable decisions. For example, investing in aluminum is a terrible investment because you could best make appropriate returns if the deliver is tight. If there is excess inside the marketplace, the expenses reduce, and therefore, you do not make sustainable earnings. In any such situation, only low-value manufacturers make earnings due to the fact they will still preserve full manufacturing, and the cycle maintains repeating itself. Opportunities to make returns best come round while the call for is extra than the manufacturing due to the growth in call for and the lower in supply. In finance, Mansharamani explains that it is made from two components; the reality fashion and the misconception. He expounds similarly using actual estates. He explains that, in fact, humans are inclined to lend and pay for the multiplied expenses. This fashion has a false impression relating to it that real property prices are not related to the willingness to lend. Moreover, when the economic establishments are open to lending, the shoppers boom, making the financial institutions to experience secure and deliver extra loans.

Feedback Loops and Equilibrium

William Lidwell & co. Defined the law of equilibrium in Universal Principles of Design. He explains that remarks is created when reactions circles returned to make an impact on themselves. In truth, all structures have a remarks loop; machines, animals, commercial enterprise, to call a few. We have two remarks loops. The tremendous remarks increases manufacturing, which in flip causes decline or boom. Contrary, bad feedback reduces manufacturing and maintains the gadget at an equilibrium point. Positive feedback brings trade and bad repercussions if the negative loop does now not modify them. For example, within the Fifties, plastic helmets with padding replaced the leather ones because of the boom in neck accidents. The helmets brought safety, but gamers until took great risks while playing, ensuing in greater neck injuries than earlier than. When designers focused on the player's behaviors, they created a fantastic loop, which made the players use their head and neck vigorously, and consequently, designers created greater plastic helmets that were more difficult and padded more. Negative feedback loops are change resisters. For example, Segway Human uses negative remarks to maintain equilibrium. When riders lean forward, it hurries up, and when the rider leans backward, it decelerates to region the system in equilibrium. To make this variation efficiently, they work towards making changes each minute.

Wait for the Regression to the Mean

Regression to the imply facilitates us to reduce judgment and cognizance on our susceptible spots in our manner of questioning. Sir Francis Galton became the first one to provide an explanation for regression to the suggest. Regression to the imply is a concept that consequences will head towards the mean as the number of effects will increase. This rule goes like trends of complicated occurrences rely upon different variables, where there is involvement of chance; average ones comply with intense outcomes. Peter Bevelin explains with an instance of John, who became no longer happy via the brand new employee's overall performance, and therefore he placed them in a application that would enhance their capabilities. They later increased their capabilities, and he concluded that this system increased made their abilities higher. Unfortunately, this isn't always the gospel fact. They would possibly have stepped forward their abilities because of regression to the imply. Since the employees have been rated as low performers, they would have improved their talents without this system, and it'd have been due to many underlying motives. Likewise, their negative competencies might had been due to exclusive reasons like fatigue, strain, or distractions. It may be that development is only a show off of their genuine capabilities.

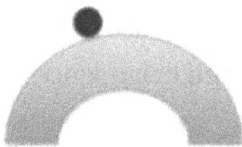

Dis-equilbrium   Equilibrium

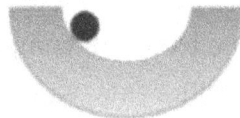

We may additionally have varied overall performance due to unique motives. Some intense performance reduces the following length because the testing measurements are by no means exact. All measurements are component real and component mistakes. If we make modifications in our mode of appearing things because of the latest unsuccessful events, we may also growth our performance the next time despite our new mode of overall performance being equal or worse. It is the principle purpose why it's miles risky to apply small samples to represent big information. It can also be the purpose James March tells us that once we live in our jobs for lengthy, the much less the distinction among the file of overall performance and the real overall performance. In regression to the imply, things maintain converting within the brief run. Its effects may be observed in sports activities in which we have unjustified speculations. Kahneman explains how a guys's ski soar, a mixture of two jumps, determines the final score. With his understanding of the regression to the imply, he wondered why the sportsman from Norway became hectic after his first amazing jump. It changed into because he hoped to protect his function or doing worse. The different sportsman from Sweden had a terrible soar before everything, and he turned into relaxed due to the fact he had nothing to lose, and this motivates him to leap better. Kahneman states that the commentator also located the regression suggest and made a tale to aid it. Our state of affairs above expounds on regression to the imply, which takes place while there's a presence of success like in our first example. Most people attach our overall performance on lack, however in fact, the technology worried is complicated, and most of what we take as being in our control are random.

Relating the imply of regression to our scenario above, a thing like wind can affect the overall performance of a jumper; if the wind is powerful, it is able to make a good athlete carry out poorly, and if the wind is favorable, a terrible jumper may additionally perform better. These results wade, and the consequences regress to the ordinary situations. Regression rule advises us to test on someone's track document when hiring as opposed to particular consequences of a state of affairs. In truth, if we've got humans inside the room who are 7 ft tall and the average height in the international is five'6''. This imply will lessen from 7 toes and get closer to the world suggest of five'6''. In the mental model, regression to the suggest ordinarily suggests up within the world of sports activities, in which we use a variety of data and numbers. In baseball, gamers can start the game batting at .500 and above, however as they keep to play greater, their average decreases to .Three hundred. Regression to the suggest also applies to gamble as nicely. A gambler will win a lot as he starts to play, however as he maintains, he loses some winnings to the house. It is how on line casino houses installation their games. Let us look at the distribution curve underneath that factors out how oftentimes an experiment will produce a positive outcome. The highest part is the average, and you could word how consequences organization round it as they growth.

https://miro.Medium.Com/max/588/1*58pAG1Ei4m4M-K8n5Uy99Q.Jpeg

What Would Bayes Do (WWBD)?

Bayes' theorem determines conditional probability. It turned into named after a well-known British mathematician Bayes Thomas.

The method above isn't always limited to finance, however it's miles significant. Baye's mental version unearths out the accuracy of medical results by way of thinking about how probably someone could have the contamination and test accuracy. In this intellectual version, we incorporate beyond chances to get future possibilities. The beyond probabilities are the chances before accumulating new data, even as future probabilities are the revised probabilities earlier than regarding new information. Statistically speaking, beyond probabilities are the probabilities of an final results with the honour that outcome B has came about. The formulation also can be used to see how the possibility of an final results is tormented by new records. For example, what is the opportunity of taking a King from a stack of cards? We have 4 kings in a fifty two playing cards percent. Therefore the possibility is 4/52, which is similar to 1/3 or 7.69%. Now, what will be the probability of having a face card? The possibility is four/12 or 33.3% because we've 12 face playing cards in a percent of playing cards.

Let us have a look at an instance of our version. We referred to that our version follows conditional opportunity, that is the opportunity of an final results on the situation that a 2nd outcome took place. We can ask ourselves what would be the opportunity of Amazon.Com discount in stock price. We can in addition ask ourselves what is going to be the opportunity of a reduction in Amazon's inventory rate with extra data that Dow Jones stock charge reduced earlier. We can express this probability as P(AMZN) because the price has decreased ad P(DJIA) because the chance of Dow Jones and the rate fell in advance. The conditional possibility might be stated as Amazon inventory fee reduces due to the earlier lower in Dow Jones, that is identical to the possibility that

Amazon fee falls and Dow Jones' falls due to the chance of a reduction in its index.

An instance of deriving Bayes' intellectual version with an example

In our formulation above, P(AMZN) and P(DJIA) are Amazon's and Dow Jones' chances without a connection. This formula explains the connection of hypothesis earlier than evidence as in Amazon's and the hypothesis after the evidence as in Dow Jones'. Let us discover more with a numerical example of the mental version.

Think of any drug test that has ninety five% accuracy. This method that this take a look at suggests ninety five% consequences on someone who is the usage of it (authentic positive) and ninety five% on someone who is not the usage of it (genuine terrible). Now, our next assumption is that only 0.6% of the population uses the drug. If you were to choose an arbitrary fine check, we ought to use the following calculations to determine if the individual is a drug user.

(zero.95 x 0.006) / [(0.95 x 0.006) + ((1- 0.95) x (1 − 0.006))] = 0.0057 / (zero.0057 + 0.0497) = 10.28%

Our version suggests that even if you examined wonderful, a non-person is much more likely to check wonderful that a user of the drug.

Chapter 7: The Map Is Not The Territory

The map of reality isn't always reality. Even the fine maps are imperfect. That's because they are discounts in what they represent. If a map were to represent the territory with perfect constancy, it'd no longer be a discount and hence might now not be beneficial to us. A map can also be a photo of a point in time, representing something that now not exists. This is important to maintain in mind as we suppose via problems and make better selections.

The Relationship Between Map And Territory

In 1931, in New Orleans, Louisiana, mathematician Alfred Korzybski presented a paper on mathematical semantics. To the non-technical reader, maximum of the paper reads like an abstruse argument on the connection of arithmetic to human language, and of both to bodily fact. Important stuff truly, but not always straight away beneficial for the layperson.

However, in his string of arguments on the shape of language, Korzybski brought and popularized the concept that the map isn't the territory. In other words, the outline of the element is not the aspect itself. The model is not fact. The abstraction isn't always abstracted. This has extensive realistic results.

Maps are important but unsuitable. (By maps, we imply any abstraction of reality, which include descriptions, theories, fashions, etc.) The problem with a map isn't always honestly that it's far an abstraction; we need abstraction. A map with a scale of 1 mile to at least one mile could no longer have the issues that maps have, nor wouldn't it be beneficial in any manner.

To solve this trouble, the thoughts creates maps of fact to be able to understand it, due to the fact the most effective manner we can method the complexity of reality is thru abstraction. But often, we don't understand our maps or their limits. In reality, we are so reliant at the abstraction that we will frequently use an wrong version without a doubt due to the fact we experience any model is most excellent to no model. (Reminding one of the under the influence of alcohol searching out his keys underneath the streetlight because "That's in which the mild is!")

Even the first-class and maximum beneficial maps be afflicted by limitations, and Korzybski offers us some to discover: (A.) The map can be wrong with out us realizing it; (B.) The map is, by means of necessity, a reduction of the actual component, a process in which you lose certain essential records; and (C.) A map needs interpretation, a manner which can motive major errors. (The best way to in reality resolve the remaining would be an limitless chain of maps-of-maps, which he called self-reflexiveness.)

With the aid of present day psychology, we also see every other problem: the human brain takes first rate leaps and shortcuts with a purpose to make sense of its surroundings. As Charlie Munger has pointed out, an amazing concept and the human thoughts act something just like the sperm and the egg — after the primary correct concept gets in, the door closes. This makes the map-territory trouble a close cousin of guy-with-a-hammer tendency.

This tendency is, manifestly, problematic in our effort to simplify fact. When we see a effective version work well, we generally tend to over-follow it, the usage of it in non-analogous situations. We have problem delimiting its usefulness, which causes mistakes.

By most accounts, Ron Johnson changed into one of the maximum successful and desirable retail executives via the summer season of 2011. Not best became he handpicked with the aid of Steve Jobs to build the Apple Stores, a undertaking which had itself come below predominant scrutiny – one retort printed in Bloomberg mag: "I deliver them two years before they're turning out the lights on a completely painful and expensive mistake" – however he have been credited with playing a primary position in turning Target from a K-Mart appearance-alike into the trendy-but-cheap Tar-they via the late Nineties and early 2000s.

Johnson's success at Apple became no longer on the spot, but it was undeniable. By 2011, Apple shops have been by using a long way the most productive in the global on a in keeping with-square-foot foundation and had end up the envy of the retail world. Their sales figures left Tiffany's inside the dirt. The sparkling glass cube on Fifth Avenue have become a greater popular visitor enchantment than the Statue of Liberty. It became a lollapalooza, something past regular fulfillment. And Johnson had led the fee.

With that fulfillment, in 2011, Johnson became hired by means of Bill Ackman, Steven Roth, and different luminaries of the monetary international to show across the dowdy old branch store chain JC Penney. The scenario of the department store changed into dour: Between 1992 and 2011, the retail marketplace proportion held by means of department shops had declined from fifty seven% to 31%.

Their middle function became a no-brainer, though. JC Penney had immensely valuable real property, anchoring shops across the u . S . A ..

Johnson argued that their bodily mall position changed into precious if for no other motive that people frequently parked next to them and walked via them to get to the center of the mall. Foot traffic became a given. Because of contracts signed inside the '50s, '60s, and '70s, the heyday of the mall constructing era, hire become also cheap, any other important competitive advantage. And not like a few suffering retailers, JC Penney become making (a few) cash. There was cash inside the check in to help fund a transformation.

The concept become to take the best ideas from his revel in at Apple, high-quality customer service, steady pricing with no markdowns and markups, immaculate displays, world-magnificence merchandise, and apply them to the department save. Johnson deliberate to turn the stores into little department stores-within-department shops. He went as far as comparing the ever-rotating shops-inside-a-store to Apple's "apps." Such a model might hold the shop continuously sparkling and avoid the creeping staleness of retail.

Johnson pitched his idea to shareholders in a sequence of ultra-modern New York City conferences paying homage to Steve Jobs' annual "But wait, there's extra!" product launches at Apple. He was persuasive: JC Penney's inventory fee went from $26 in the summer time of 2011 to $42 in early 2012 on the electricity of the pitch.

The idea failed almost at once. His new pricing version (disposing of discounting) was a flop. The coupon-hunters rebelled. Much of his new product become deemed too modern day. His new shop version was wildly high-priced for a middling branch shop chain – including running losses purposefully persisted, and he'd spent numerous billion bucks looking to impact the bodily transformation of the shops. JC Penney customers had no idea what turned into taking place, and via 2013, Johnson turned into sacked. The inventory charge sank into the unmarried digits, in which it stays two years later.

What went wrong inside the quest to build America's Favorite Store? It became out that

Johnson became using a map of Tulsa to navigate Tuscaloosa. Apple's merchandise, customers, and history had far too little in common with JC Penney's. Apple had a rabid, younger, affluent fan-base before they built stores; JC Penney's become not associated with young people or affluence. Apple had shiny merchandise, and wished a shiny keep; JC Penney changed into recognised for its affordable sweaters. Apple had never relied on discounting inside the first place; JC Penney became removing reductions given prior, triggering big deprival superb-reaction.

In different words, the antique map turned into not very beneficial. Even his achievement at Target, which looks like a more in-depth analog, changed into deceptive in the context of JC Penney. Target had made small, incremental modifications over many years, to which Johnson had made a significant contribution. JC Penney became attempting to reinvent the concept of the department shop in a yr or two, leaving in the back of the center purchaser in an attempt to advantage new ones. This became a miles distinct proposition. (Another aspect retaining the corporation back changed into surely its base odds: Can you name a store of superb significance that has misplaced its role in the international and are available again?)

The predominant issue changed into now not that Johnson become incompetent. He wasn't. He wouldn't are becoming the task if he turned into. He turned into extremely ready. But it changed into precisely his competence and beyond success that were given him into problem. He was like a tremendous swimmer that attempted to address a grand fast, and the version he used correctly in the past, the map that had navigated lots of tough terrains, turned into not the map he wanted anymore. He had an great theory about retailing that implemented in some occasions, but no longer in others. The terrain had changed, but the antique idea caught.

Taleb has been vocal about the misuse of models for many years, but the earliest and most bright I can recall is his company grievance of a monetary model called Value-at-Risk, or VAR. The model, used within the banking network, is supposed to assist manipulate hazard by means of providing a most potential loss inside a given self assurance c program languageperiod. In different phrases, it purports to allow threat managers to say that, within ninety five%, 99%, or ninety nine.9% self assurance, the company will no longer lose greater than $X million dollars on a given day. The better the c language, the less correct the evaluation turns into. It is probably possible to mention that the corporation has $one hundred million at threat at any time at a ninety nine% self belief c language, but given the statistical properties of markets, a pass to 99.Nine% confidence might mean the danger manager has to nation the company has $1 billion at danger. 99.Ninety nine% would possibly suggest $10 billion. As rarer and rarer activities are covered within the distribution, the analysis gets less beneficial. So, by means of necessity, the "tails" are cut off someplace, and the evaluation is deemed proper.

Elaborate statistical fashions are constructed to justify and use the VAR concept. On its face, it seems like a beneficial and effective idea; in case you recognize how much you may lose at any time, you may manage threat to the decimal. You can inform your board of administrators and shareholders, with a instantly face, which you've got your eye on the till.

In order to give you the VAR figure, the danger manager must take ancient records and assume a statistical distribution if you want to are expecting the future. For instance, if we may want to take one hundred million humans and examine their height and weight, we could then predict the distribution of heights and weights on a exceptional one hundred million, and there might be a microscopically small opportunity that we'd be incorrect. That's because we've got a massive sample size, and we're studying something with very small and predictable deviations from the average.

But finance does no longer follow this type of distribution. There's no such predictability. As Nassim has argued, the "tails" are fats on this area, and the rarest, most unpredictable activities have the biggest consequences. Let's say you deem a highly threatening occasion (for instance, a ninety% crash within the S&P 500) to have a 1 in 10,000 chance of happening in a given yr, and your historical information set simplest has 300 years of information. How are you able to appropriately state the probability of that event? You would want a long way more data.

Thus, monetary activities deemed to be five, or 6, or 7 fashionable deviations from the norm tend to occur with a certain regularity that nowhere near suits their intended statistical possibility. Financial markets don't have any organic truth to tie them down: We can say with a useful amount of self belief that an elephant will not wake up as a monkey, but we can't say some thing with no question in an Extremistan area.

We see numerous issues with VAR as a "map," then. The first that the version is itself a extreme abstraction of reality, counting on ancient facts to predict the destiny. (As all financial fashions must, to a positive volume.) VAR does now not say, "The danger of dropping

X dollars is Y, within a self assurance of Z." (Although threat managers deal with it that way). What VAR sincerely says is, "the threat of losing X greenbacks is Y, based at the given parameters." The hassle is apparent even to the non-technician: The destiny is a abnormal and foreign region that we do now not recognize. Deviations of the beyond might not be the deviations of the destiny. Just due to the fact municipal bonds have never traded at such-and-this type of spread to U.S. Treasury bonds does no longer suggest that they received't paintings within the future. They just haven't but. Frequently, the fashions are unaware of this reality.

In truth, one of Nassim's maximum trenchant factors is that at the day before, anything "worst-case" occasion occurred in the past, you'll no longer have been using the coming "worst case" as your worst case, as it wouldn't have took place yet.

Here's an easy example. On October 19, 1987, the inventory market dropped with the aid of 22.Sixty one% or 508 points at the Dow Jones

Industrial Average. In percentage terms, it became then and remained the worst one-day marketplace drop in U.S. History. It was dubbed "Black Monday." (Financial writers every now and then lack creativity — there are several other "Black Mondays" in history.) But right here we see Nassim's point: On October 18, 1987, what would the models use because the worst possible case? We don't know precisely, however we do recognise the preceding worst case become 12.82%, which came about on October 28, 1929. A 22.61% drop would have been taken into consideration such a lot of fashionable deviations from the average as to be near impossible.

But the tails are very fat in finance — improbable and consequential occasions appear to appear a ways greater frequently than they should be primarily based on naive facts. There is likewise a excessive however often unrecognized recursiveness hassle, that's that the fashions themselves have an impact on the final results they are looking to predict.

This is sort of a GPS gadget that shows you where you're at all times however doesn't include cliffs. You'd be perfectly happy together with your GPS till you drove off a mountain.

It became this kind of naive consider of models that got a whole lot of human beings in trouble within the latest mortgage crisis. Backward-looking, trend-becoming fashions, the most not unusual maps of the financial territory, failed via describing a territory that became best a mirage: A global where home costs only went up.

The logical reaction to all this is, "So what?" If our maps fail us, how will we perform in an uncertain world? This is its very own dialogue for over again, and Taleb has gone to great pains to try and address the concern. Smart minds disagree on the solution. But one obvious key ought to be constructing structures that are robust to version error.

The practical hassle with a version like VAR is that the banks use it to optimize. In different words, they take on as a good deal publicity as the version deems OK. And whilst banks veer into dealing with to a fantastically unique, exceptionally confident version in place of to informed common feel, which happens often, they tend to accumulate hidden dangers in an effort to un-disguise themselves in time.

If one were to instead expect that there have been no precisely accurate maps of the monetary territory, they could have to fall back on an awful lot less complicated heuristics. (If you anticipate special statistical fashions of the destiny will fail you, you don't use them.)

In brief, you would do what Warren Buffett has done with Berkshire Hathaway. Mr. Buffett, to our know-how, has never used a computer model in his existence, but manages an group 1/2 one trillion bucks in length by using property, a large part of which can be economic assets. How?

The approach calls for not simplest assuming a destiny worst-case some distance greater extreme than the beyond, but additionally dictates constructing an group with a sturdy set of backup systems, and margins-of-safety operating at multiple levels. Extra cash, as opposed to greater leverage. Taking fantastic pains to make certain the tails can't kill you, as opposed to optimizing to a version, accepting the limits of your clairvoyance.

The salient point then is that during our march to simplify fact with beneficial fashions, of which Farnam Street is an recommend, we confuse the models with fact. For many humans, the version creates its own fact. It is as though the spreadsheet involves existence. We neglect that fact is lots messier. The map isn't the territory. The theory isn't what it describes; it's absolutely a way we choose to interpret a sure set of statistics. Maps can also be wrong, but even supposing they may be essentially accurate, they're an abstraction, and abstraction means that records is misplaced to store area. (Recall the mile-to-mile scale map.)

Chapter 8: The Origin Of Mental Models

As we've got visible, our intellectual models emerge lengthy earlier than we're born. Culturally speaking, its beginning factors to loads or maybe thousands of years earlier than us. But over time, our organic barriers, our non-public history, and our appropriation via the specific kinds of language will manual the way we assume and act. It is from this combination of factors that we build and corporation opinions. More crucial than understanding the foundation of those mental fashions, is making an attempt to take the reins on them. Not to be over excited with the aid of the automatism of preconceived concepts is the primary mission of the recurring. After all, it is not because you have usually understood a subject in a sure manner that desires to go on like this.

Mental Models That Block Creativity

"I can't do it." "I do not have the potential." "I will no longer strive because it will now not paintings."

These are typical phrases that we repeat in hard conditions that require going beyond the normal. But maybe it is time you re-idea the use of every phrase and line you talk. The human unconscious once in a while imposes obstacles on our actions. These are the so-referred to as proscribing mind, which make us fear new and one-of-a-kind reports. It is that kind of reasoning that most effective results in the not unusual and stops something innovative from being externalized. Do you realize the ones conventional terms, the clichés like "each flesh presser is a thief" or "blonde is dumb"?

The point right here is to go away such expressions apart and permit your self to head similarly, to recognize the meaning behind every story and no longer simply repeat what most propagates as truth.

Discover your Mental Models

You may also recognize the origin of your mental models, however have you ever stopped to surprise why they affect you in a sure manner? Trying to discover, in truth, what these patterns are and to recognize what they mean is a way to appropriate even more of your mind and feelings.

Want to apprehend how? Check out the following recommendations which I have collated and listed beneath:

Self

The first query you need to ask your self is: do I virtually recognise myself?

Looking at your self and seeking answers is the first step in expertise the way you relate to people and the world. Aggression, for example, is a reasonably not unusual feeling amongst folks that attempt only to stifle the struggles they day by day struggle within to discover what they count on from lifestyles.

Empathy

As you begin to exercise self-knowledge and recognize your own doubts, it turns into an awful lot less difficult to relate to the outdoor international. This additionally method exercising empathy. The easy workout of setting oneself within the other's region opens up a universe of infinite opportunities of know-how. You will see that your colleague's mind-set turned into based totally on his four assets and filters, which can be absolutely distinct from yours.

Respect

After all, the herbal way is that of recognize for contrary evaluations. But this is also an exercise you have to result in. Each man or woman has his/her very own intellectual version, made out of their personal, cultural, and other reports - and there may be not anything wrong with it. The crucial component is not to make it the most effective option.

By performing those sports, you will be tons toward discovering and controlling your personal idea styles. Now, I am guessing that the subsequent query might be the logically subsequent query in your thoughts:

How to Make Use of Knowledge?

In order for our fashions now not to close in on themselves, we have to always be looking for expertise. It's now not due to the fact some thing labored twenty years ago, so it will constantly be the fine opportunity. This manner our mental fashions need to be elevated.

Do you understand that infant's toy wherein every geometrical parent need to be positioned in the area corresponding to its design? Our mental fashions work in a similar way. And no, I am no longer joking.

Your experience handiest gave you the reading of a circle. However, the moment offers you a rectangular. The simplest can also appear to cut the rims of the square so that it serves in the area of the sector, however someone who adapts and seeks know-how will try to recognize the reading of the parent and what lies behind it.

Mental models are all about control. It is not hard to look again and remember large brands which have failed or misplaced their marketplace space. Accustomed to a distinct global, they were no longer able to adapt to cultural and technological modifications.

That is, based totally on their very own intellectual fashions, the managers did no longer recognize that the transformation was a simple circumstance for the employer to retain occupying its space. And startups quick occupied these gaps, which had been ready to be filled. It is something that can't be unnoticed.

The Influence of Mental Models on Corporate Results

The fulfillment story of Southwest Airlines, a Texan airline, shows what we have just stated. The agency, which has massive competition inclusive of Delta and United, is the simplest one inside the industry to make a income for forty three consecutive years. This is because, when you consider that its basis, it has an open intellectual version that permits figuring out market developments.

While the other organizations are making an investment in trendy aircraft, with class A, B, C and D cabins and multi-stop flights, Southwest has more modest plane fashions without stipulating socioeconomic divisions for passengers and non-prevent journey. This is a sort of commercial enterprise that grew out of the belief that there was a particular client who had buying strength however not sufficient to pay for all the luxuries of an air ride.

Looking at the carrier in a one of a kind manner made it feasible to enter a segment that had no longer been explored till then. Hence, you may ask, "Oh, however have not competition tried to repeat the business model?" They attempted, however they did no longer have the same fulfillment as we noted earlier than. This occurred because the public did not purchase the idea and preferred to maintain flying with the employer that from the beginning, was dedicated to it.

How Does The Mental Model Of Leaders Impact On Company Performance?

Believe it or not, intellectual fashions of leaders do impact business enterprise overall performance plenty. Any and each decision made by using a organisation's leaders is in some manner primarily based on their intellectual models. That is, the effect is direct and looks in each of the alternatives made.

Mental Models in Leadership

Want a nice instance of a intellectual model of a very good chief? He is the one who takes obligation and does now not blame each person. This kind of manager is proactive and shares his accomplishments with the crew. When he realizes that something is incorrect, he attempts to discover a solution, rather than simply stating the trouble. It is someone who allows resolve conflicts and seeks to listen what others have to say. If you want to observe the version of an excellent leader, this is the way.

Brief Conclusion

Mental models are gift at some point of our lives, and they start present considering that even before we have been born. As a great deal as you would possibly try to forget about them, they'll seem on your choices. They are so natural that we often do not even word it.

The important factor is to realize the way to use them in our desire, in a manner that affects our moves positively. To get there, bear in mind these 3 phrases: self-know-how, empathy, and recognize.

Understanding the intellectual models which might be a part of your existence is fundamental to know-how human conduct as well. In reality, intellectual models can decide a person's achievement or failure. I even have lengthy wanted to write a e-book or some thing else about mental models, as a good deal as I like the problem. When I ask absolutely everyone I talk to on the topic or maybe in any other case as to what this indicates, some humans take a look at me apprehensively and are waiting for a tip, however the question is mine, and I constantly try to extract the answer in keeping with the general information of the institution. When you apprehend the idea and are seeking to associate it in exercise, the adventure turns into much less painful.

Understanding the premise of human conduct and the keys to private achievement depends on information the that means and importance of mental fashions in your lifestyles. Whether you are aware of it or not, mental fashions outline your potential to act and react to the simplest things and the hardest matters in life; this is, they define your conduct.

First, it's miles important to recognise the assets of mental models and the way they are fashioned. According to Daniel Goleman, writer of the bestselling e-book referred to as Emotional Intelligence, the assets of intellectual fashions are the way humans arrange and provide that means to their reviews. According to Goleman, human conduct is conditioned by using mental fashions, and those, in flip, are described based totally on 4 assumptions:

Biology: labeling the human being's capability to carry out primarily based on its physiological barriers. Does the reality that someone is tall or short, black or white, hairy or bald, fats or thin, lovely or less preferred in phrases of beauty, should be a thing of inclusion or exclusion within the task marketplace? For many companies, this is the way it works, lamentably. Have you ever study a task advertisement within the newspaper with the following words:

Do you need a Chubby Secretary, quick, and the whole thing which greater or much less approach something about the advent and much less approximately the abilties or intelligence?

Language: is the medium wherein the consciousness of the individual is established. When you hear a Northeasterner, a Santa Catarina, a gaucho from the pampas, a Paulista from the interior or a carioca with a verbal exchange with that standard accent of his place, what comes for your mind? Do no longer say you've got never categorized someone because of your accessory? Enjoy! But baaah !!!

Culture: within any group - households, industries, groups, and nations - collective intellectual models increase from shared studies. Thus tradition can be considered a collective intellectual model. If you are the child of Jew, Italian, Greek, German, or Japanese, it does now not matter, and there's a hard and fast of values or assumptions typical of each lifestyle. Somehow this affects relationships, subsequently the problems of admitting in a few cultures the union of human beings from exclusive roots.

Personal enjoy: concerns race, gender, nationality, ethnic foundation, social and economic circumstance, circle of relatives influences, degree of education, how we had been handled by way of our parents, siblings, teachers and youth companions. The way we begin to work and acquire self-sufficiency is also the fruit of our private experience, and this is key to our achievement.

Because of all this, some phrases end up not unusual in your every day existence and when you least count on it, inadvertently slip, without the least subject for the reflection of your phrases. What counts for one us of a or culture isn't always always legitimate for any other. Have you ever uttered any of those terms?

All men are equal! It manner that your father and that man or woman you both recognize are also. You can not trust ladies! Even your mom, your spouse, and your sisters?

All politicians are identical! Including that his relative who were very difficult-fought and determined a task for his entire own family that was in hassle?

The little with God is enough! Believe me, if this is authentic, the most you will reap is without a doubt that 'little,' and on the identical time, you may continue to envy the rich for the rest of your lifestyles.

This isn't going to paintings, and it has constantly been like this right here! This is one of the maximum famous mental fashions in agencies that are doomed to fail.

I'm terrible, however I'm satisfied! Do you recognize a few terrible, inside the literal sense of the word, happy?

The important aspect is to win! More important than prevailing is contributing and not being overwhelmed via defeat. If the world were made handiest of victors, mastering might no longer exist.

These are a number of the hundreds of mental fashions established based on our biology, language, tradition, and private experience. When taken actually, mental models are capable of inflicting actual havoc in our private and professional lives. However, you have to no longer ignore them, just be careful to avoid prejudices designed solely on the premise of values that may be part of one subculture and no longer any other.

For FredyKofman, writer of Metamanagement, the mental model is the set of meanings, assumptions, policies of reasoning, inferences, and so forth, which leads us to make a positive interpretation. They define how we perceive, sense, assume, and have interaction. Therefore, it is fundamental to immerse ourselves in extraordinary cultures, disciplines, studies, and languages with out dropping our origins.

All cultures have some thing to educate approximately human conduct from special angles of imaginative and prescient; just realize how to respect them. The Jewish maxim expressed inside the Talmud helps us higher recognize this reasoning: "We do no longer see matters as they may be, we see things as we are." Think about it and be satisfied!

Chapter 9: Knowing When Mental Models Have Outlived Their Usefulness

Mental models come to be a effective tool when a person learns to perceive them and observe them to issues and choices. However, it is not unusual for humans to keep onto mental models which are now not beneficial. For instance, the Atlantic slave trade ended over one hundred years ago. Even so, the devastating consequences have left the whole area on protect. People are nonetheless cautious these days due to the fact they were taught to remain careful and on protect.

Before you may conquer inaccurate mental fashions or mental fashions which have outlived their usefulness, you'll must become aware of them. This may be a venture, as many people have a mental block against those matters that disprove their middle ideals. This chapter will go over some of the ways that mental models can be incorrect, so that you can extra severely evaluate which mental models to preserve, which to construct on, and which to replace with greater effective models.

Attention and Perception

Mental models have an effect on recognition. As cited earlier, Warren Buffett and Charlie Munger look for positive indicators that tell them a enterprise has a threat of boom before making an funding. However, this cognizance manner that they do no longer consciousness on other areas of the enterprise and there is a few danger of overlooking facts.

Mental models affect what a person chooses to pay attention to and the way they perceive the information they have got available. It can even have an effect on the facts this is with no trouble to be had within the mind. Additionally, many people fill in information this is regular with whatever mental version they are maximum familiar with. For instance, a person who has a popular mistrust for leaders or political participants as being untrustworthy is much more likely to accumulate statistics and use it to deduce that a leader is appearing unethically instead of to evaluate their politics.

They may additionally even take the records amassed and re-examine it, actively running to stay steady with that category (untrustworthiness) that they relate to political figures.

Breaking Traditions

Many beliefs cannot be examined on my own, as lots of humans's beliefs are exceeded down by popular society. For instance, it became many years before countries common that human beings of African American descent could be right leaders. Likewise, women are not closely concerned at an higher leadership degree due to the fact now not all of society believes a female is capable of leading. To disprove this idea, however, it should be examined on the societal level.

Societal ideals trickle down through generations. When a parent does now not believe the authorities, this same mistrust regularly trickles down thru the generations. Even even though kids are unfastened to pick out their personal ideals, their parental affect could make it impossible for them to check this distrust at a societal stage till many others are geared up to test that belief. This is one of the motives that it's miles considered such a feat when a country has its first lady leader or their first coloured leader—it represents a shift in the attitudes through the complete united states of america and a technology that is extra accepting of trade and the possibility that the mental models they've believed most in their lives need to be challenged.

Belief Traps

When a person believes some thing, it creates what's called a perception lure. This trap prevents theories from ever being examined due to the fact the man or woman believes their mental version on the sort of deep stage. For example, after an financial disintegrate, human beings can be much less in all likelihood to put cash in a bank or rely on a financial institution. Even years after the initial event, this distrust can also continue to be and a person may keep heading off running with economic establishments. There is always a chance that they might work with the banks once more and have remarkable benefits, renewing their consider, however a few people will not take that hazard. People are certainly inclined to do the ones matters that they're comfortable with instead of trying out new waters.

As the stakes get better, the chance that someone will take the threat of challenging their mental model decreases. For example, there are medical practices like genital mutilation which might be usually disapproved by using advanced nations. However, a few nations tell moms that failing to have a lady's genitals mutilated can lower the risk of fertility or that it could be dangerous or fatal in some way if the system isn't done. Even although we realize within the evolved global that the exercise is barbaric, it takes a brave mom to mission the concept and risk harm to her woman child. Another bizarre dependancy practiced in some international locations is enamel extraction for newborns wherein undeveloped infant enamel are removed to keep away from contamination or sickness.

Parents regularly do no longer believe they have the capacity to mission docs—they simply want their infant to get higher and there may be an expert telling them that is the way. Additionally, there may be the chance (and guilt) associated with forgoing the clinical process and risking something occurring to their toddler or their toddler's infection getting worse. Even though there will be a exceptional praise (heading off a painful and pointless clinical method), this comes with first rate hazard.

Confirmation Bias and Ideology

Nobody likes to be advised they are wrong. The human ego regularly interacts with the mind in a way that makes people suppress, neglect, or forget about any observations that don't align with their core ideologies. Likewise, affirmation bias reasons people to search for and use that statistics that supports their own core beliefs, as opposed to seeking out balanced or new data that might show the contrary.

The human tendency to dismiss new and useful information in light of last 'proper' of their beliefs is a main roadblock to fulfillment. Think of it this manner—are you successful on your existence proper now? As a hit as you need to be? Odds are, you continue to have desires that you want to reach and different things to do before you acquire fulfillment, whether at paintings or to your non-public life. This model of success cannot be added about with out trade. To alternate, human beings must be inclined to accept new records and observe it seriously, instead of allow bias to don't forget tainting their view of the arena.

Additionally, a few people war with affirmation bias due to the fact they have no longer shared the enjoy of a person else. For instance, within the United States, sexual harassment is a problem within the place of business. Even so, many girls do no longer communicate up because they are afraid of dropping their jobs, not being believed by way of preferred society, or other effects. This happens due to the fact as a whole, society is made to believe that sexual harassment is not a hassle and the ladies who do revel in it is outliers. When women percentage their experiences, others have trouble knowledge them or accepting that communication. Therefore, the female does no longer have her worries verified and the unfairness keeps on.

Changing Mental Models on a Larger Level

One of the biggest obstacles whilst using mental models to interpret the sector for a positive purpose is that the arena and societal views deeply affect mental models, mainly across gender and social castes. In Malawi, as an example, it is not unusual for women farmers to be disregarded while they convey their thoughts ahead, as they may be considered much less informed than guys even though they have the identical information base. This takes place in India too, whilst even educated ladies are taken into consideration much less credible than their male counterparts.

On the other aspect, government regulations can assist shift public attitudes away from problems derived from stereotypes. For example, even after slavery ended inside the United States, segregation remained a problem till it turned into removed. Even after the regulations, but, there was an obstacle inside the mental models and fashionable poor mindset that a few human beings hold to have in the direction of human beings of a exclusive skin shade. This isn't something based totally on reality in most cases, only a concept that has been handed down without being challenged via generations of people. The chance that someone could have racist ideals is more potent in positive regions. However, this more than probable stems from the reality that folks that like those who they see as just like them. When they permit a person's skin color to steer their opinion greater than someone's persona, they are proscribing themselves via failing to word the obvious similarities that all of us percentage as human beings.

Of route, regulations change as attitudes shift. These guidelines can come from a government stage however can also be prompted by the media. In India, as an example, policies have shifted the manner that girls are treated in politics. In West Bengal, but, one village created a political affirmative action for women that allowed them the opportunity t lead for the first time. As this become implemented across distinct villages, it brought about extra girls main. After seven years, male attitudes have been re-evaluated to peer if they had shifted. Even although guys still had a desire of male to woman leaders, they had been assured via lady leaders who met certain requirements and had been considered ready leaders. In addition to influencing the manner men considered ladies leaders, the change in policy (and intellectual models) shifted society as an entire. Parents had new aspirations for their teenage daughters, adolescent girls had a better aspiration for themselves, and the gender hole in schooling in India narrowed barely.

Even although the case in India represents a superb prevalence, regrettably, the coverage does no longer usually take preserve this manner. In any other village in India, political affirmative motion turned into used to encourage teachers with a decrease social repute to run for village authorities. Unfortunately, this had the terrible effect of growing absenteeism in better-caste teachers, which also expanded terrible effects in village schools. This turned into delivered approximately via the resistance from high-caste instructors as they resisted the exchange that turned into being added approximately.

The media can also affect a person's mental models. For instance, overpopulation is a problem in many nations. More than probably, this fashion comes from excessive start prices from families that follow the cultural tradition of getting large households with many kids. The have a look at increased exposure to the concept by means of exposing groups to particularly attractive cleaning soap operas. These soap operas had been focused heavily on households with fewer children. Over the years, fertility fees declined. This identical technique turned into carried out across many municipalities in Brazil, efficiently decreasing fertility rates.

One of the most influential techniques of converting mental models is early youth intervention. Studies have shown that the schooling gadget may be used to shape a child's perspectives on the world. For instance, while children are endorsed to engage in classroom discussions and interact with classmates and their trainer, it can growth their level of accept as true with, mainly for people in their social organization.

How to Change Your Personal Mental Models

As you study greater about the ones mental models in your existence that no longer serve you, it's miles essential to continue developing your collection and including the ones models that provide advantages. The first step is tough the ones intellectual models that do not serve you. Even even though racism is typically accepted as incorrect, folks who had been raised through racist dad and mom have greater problem overcoming their aversion to human beings of a extraordinary pores and skin color.

The key to converting intellectual fashions that do not serve you is beginning at a special point inside the system. Often, the intellectual fashions which can be maximum damaging are those which are prompted right away and motive motion. Every choice goes via a cycle that consists of:

Taking moves that align with your beliefs

Adopting ideals approximately the arena

Drawing conclusions

Making assumptions in line with which means

Adding non-public and cultural meanings to statistics

Selection discovered information

·Observing reports and facts

This cycle is a regular loop. Many human beings cope with their intellectual models on the top, where they have already been stimulated to action. However, it is simplest to jump into this loop at the bottom. Here, whilst you are watching data and studies, you have got the energy to consciously exchange what you take note of. Instead of quick assigning information to what you're seeing and experiencing, it is vital to take a step returned and observe it from every other angle. Then, you could use the new facts to incite exchange.

There are several methods to break this cycle. You can:

Be privy to mind and possible fallacies in reasoning by means of asking questions about our personal beliefs

Use examples, information, and records accumulating to guide a more recent, more desirable mental version

Ask approximately others' thinking and challenge our very own point of view

Interpret meaning for ourselves as opposed to making assumptions

·Align thoughts with our middle ideals and self-expression

You need to never be afraid to question your beliefs. In fact, questioning beliefs is one detail that can help you overcome your ideals. Find out if what you accept as true with is based on truth or assumption. Then, allow your internal communicate to help you address complicated troubles. It can also be beneficial to speak with a person else who has distinct core beliefs, particularly once you are open to a new way of thinking and willing to listen to their specific attitude. Then, make an effort to mirror for your thoughts, emotions, and behaviors. As you realise the relationship among this stuff, you'll study the consequences of your thoughts, emotions, and behaviors in your personal instances and the sector around you.

Once you've got standard that a mental version now not serves you, it's going to take time to conquer your initial assumptions. When you are making selections or resolve issues, take the time to be sure those assumptions aren't affecting your ability to have clean mind. It will take conscious effort for some time and cautious assessment of your thoughts. As you still consciously refute the undesirable mental version and disprove it, your mind will notice your efforts and ultimately trade that pathway of wondering.

Chapter 10: The Decision-Making Process

From the instant we awaken inside the morning we're faced with selections to make. What to put on, which path to take to the office, what to consume, who to name and so on and so forth. It is a never-finishing move of alternatives that we need to make to determine how our day will pass. The cumulative effect of those little choices and the big selections that we make automatically is what shapes our conduct and in the long run the route of our lives.

Think of a woman who takes an unplanned stroll outside their everyday habitual and bumps into the stranger who later becomes their spouse or the internet entrepreneur who at some point walked out of a literature magnificence in university and decided to start a YouTube channel. These incidences occur to humans every day. A reputedly trivial choice can modify the course of your existence or alternate your outcome extensively.

The trouble in decision making is that irrespective of how careful we're it is not usually possible to are expecting the destiny. We can also make cautious selections to keep away from bad effects however in the long run the destiny is unknown or even good selections can now and again bring about terrible results. Focusing too much on the preferred outcome way that we ignore the procedure, make assumptions and leap to conclusions with a view to arrive on the favored final results quicker.

The secret to meaking selections is developing a sound decision-making manner this is built on an goal idea method and rational observations. Achieving goals, enjoyable life long dreams and establishing exact relationships all take time, power and effort or even with a lot of these we cannot assure a successful final results.

A private failure like achievement is a natural part of the human enjoy. To keep away from indecision and procrastination you need to be able to make selections even with the expertise that there's usually a opportunity which you may fail. The fear of failure makes us remove decisions due to the fact we are terrified of making a mistake or getting a bad final results. Procrastination results in state of no activity. While you can fail if you strive, you're assured to fail in case you don't attempt.

To be proactive and to keep away from inertia or stalling, while faced with vital decisions it's far important to don't forget that the decision-making method is as important because the result itself because it results in motion.

Mental Models and Thinking

Our belief of humans, situations, and experiences in addition to our interpretation of the world around us is executed via the intellectual models we create. Mental fashions form our notion processes and in turn affect our moves and conduct. We generally tend to make decisions primarily based on our ideals, options, and reviews, no longer simply logic alone. This method that emotions and individual biases often influence our decision-making system and this effects in impaired judgment and terrible decision making.

Understanding exclusive intellectual models can deliver us an information of ways our thought technique happens when it comes to our perception, feelings, and ideals. Our belief and belief structures range from person to man or woman because we each have our own precise reviews and techniques of filtering expertise that form how we view systems and occurrences.

We tend to understand situations in a way that enhances our beliefs and conforms to the assumptions we've got evolved through the years. This can supply us a fake experience of reality with the aid of developing a reality this is tainted with our biases and options. Any new information and statistics that we collect are filtered through the intellectual fashions we've created and advanced in our minds.

The intellectual fashions at our disposal when it comes to questioning play a main function in simplifying complex systems into easy ideas that we will apprehend, give an explanation for and make use of. Our choice-making manner is greater greatly by means of having numerous and interdisciplinary mental models through which we will organize and examine statistics.

To apprehend the role of intellectual models in our questioning technique we ought to understand their predominant traits which might be;

They are incomplete in their representation of the sector and are constantly changing and evolving with enjoy and gaining knowledge of.

They are not actual representations of reality however are as an alternative are individual interpretations of truth.

They simplify complicated know-how and reviews by using organizing information. Into easy concepts that we are able to apprehend.

·Each version is a representation of a probable outcome

Our exceptional of concept and potential to make precise decisions is determined to a massive volume through the range of intellectual models we've in our minds and their variety of utility. Having a mental version gives us with a machine via which we are able to filter records and recognize the complex structures and conditions.

Mental fashions are gear in our mental toolboxes that we will use in making choices, generating ideas and fixing issues. Using this analogy, it's miles clean that the greater intellectual fashions you've got at your disposal the more your variety and intensity of mind and in effect the greater conditions and troubles you will be able to take care of.

Over-dependence on a limited quantity of intellectual models restricts us to just a slim view of the arena that will be primarily based on our beliefs and prejudices. In the identical way that seeing out of 1 eye might be possible however limiting in phrases of the sector of imaginative and prescient, the use of a restricted set of mental fashions is also feasible but confines your thoughts to a fixed pattern ensuing in patterns of behavior that grow to be normal.

For innovation and ideas to be generated we ought to find new ways of thinking and interpreting information. Thinking as you have always done, in the equal styles of thought, is sure to offer you the equal results you've got usually gotten. Change in our lives starts offevolved with the alternate in our thoughts and the handiest manner to correctly alternate our mind is by means of constantly obtaining new intellectual models.

Perception

Perception is a center detail inside the formation of mental models. Our experience of the world round and the diverse phenomena we engage with is interpreted thru perception. Perception includes the recognition of external stimuli and the reactions that occur in reaction to that stimuli. We use the notion manner to benefit an expertise of the one-of-a-kind structures that we come into touch with.

Perception is the idea via which we form a courting with various structures and with the arena round us in preferred. Perception offers us a guideline on how to relate to the specific systems we automatically have interaction with. Perception takes place in a sequence of distinct processes.

The first level within the belief method is publicity to stimuli which takes place mechanically as we engage with different systems in our immediate environment. This interaction can occur through either of our five senses, sight, contact, sound, scent and flavor. Once we're exposed to the stimuli, our mind is going to paintings decoding and figuring out the stimulus. Once we have identified it, we are able to then react accurately to it.

This technique takes place clearly and constantly. We are surrounded by one of a kind styles of stimuli that appeal to our interest in some unspecified time in the future or the. These stimuli encompass whatever that may be touched, heard, seen, tasted, or smelled. The particular stimulus that draws our attention will become the attended stimulus. The attended stimulus is then transmitted as a neuro signal to the brain. Once it reaches the mind, we then end up consciously privy to the presence of the stimulus within the environment.

The diagnosed stimulus is then categorized and identified. Once the stimulus has been identified we can then act in the proper way in response to the perceived stimulus. Our belief we will for that reason surmise is built on 4 main elements;

1.Receiving statistics or information.

2.Selection of facts based totally on external or inner factors.

three.Organization of the statistics into standards.

four.Interpretation of the facts to elicit a response.

To understand and make feel of the sector, we absorb power from the surroundings and convert it to neuro signals; that is the technique of sensation. Perception can occur in wonderful pathways. The kind of belief that happens in a bottom-up sequence of processing of stimulus starts offevolved with the stimulus and ends with the identification and categorization of that stimulus.

In to- down processing form of belief, the notion is evolved based totally on beyond enjoy and our expectations. Data, in this example, is interpreted on the basis of the context wherein the stimulus happens or exists. The top-down processing series of notion happens whilst we start with a larger object and then gather more data at the object in query.

In pinnacle-down processing of perception, we begin with a standard concept then progressively damage it all the way down to more exact smaller ideas. Top-down processing facilitates in simplifying our view of the world, through taking in data in vast generalized impressions in preference to having to consciousness on multiple small remoted information. Top-down processing is conceptually driven. It is influenced by using expectancies, existing ideals and our know-how of numerous structures.

The pinnacle-down processing of perceived stimulus is beneficial while seeking out patterns in the surroundings however it is able to confine us to a fixed and stuck way of perceiving things due to the fact we rely on beyond experience to make inferences. The context and situations in which an item is perceived can affect our expectations. The foremost Influences that affect our notion encompass;

Past studies

Assumptions and expectancies.

Education

Values and beliefs

·Circumstances

All those impacts predispose us to awareness on sure statistics that confirms our ideals and discounting the records that goes towards those beliefs. We assemble our personal belief based totally on how we select to look and interpret the sector round us. In the cease, belief performs a massive role in how we suppose, act and behave.

Emotions

Good selections require that an individual be self-conscious, able to manipulate their feelings and have the ability to narrate their feelings to knowledge if you want to make sound choices. The growing awareness on emotional intelligence is an acknowledgment of the crucial function it performs in non-public fulfillment in addition to in creating cohesive and efficient societies.

Developing and preserving intellectual fashions for effective questioning and choice-making techniques calls for emotional intelligence. Emotional intelligence is the capacity to understand and control our very own emotions as well as the ones of the human beings around us.

From the instant we awaken in the morning, we start to experience feelings based totally on what we are questioning and our present instances. Emotions will have a extensive effect on our choice-making method and notion system. Salesmen play on our feelings to get us to shop for things we might not actually need.

Thousands of advertising campaigns and advertisements target our emotional reactions through developing commercials that tug at our heartstrings and activate us to create a wonderful association for the product being advertised. The power of emotions over our decisions is deep and a ways-attaining. Without self-recognition and strength of will, we end up predisposed to creating decisions primarily based on how we sense rather than basing selections on logic.

Emotional have an effect on on our concept processes, conduct and actions is the purpose self-attention and self-regulation are the middle factors required to achieve emotional intelligence. When we allow bad feelings to modify our actions and conduct, we become affecting our overall performance, objectivity and the clarity of notion required to make sound selections. When we feature forward bad feelings from beyond experiences, it impacts how we behave inside the gift and diminishes largely our ability to create a tremendous future.

Emotional intelligence is a core competence in all spheres of lifestyles including private existence, social interactions, and career improvement. Developing and improving our EQ must, therefore, be a constant and non-stop enterprise to help us achieve a satisfied, fulfilled and efficient lifestyles. Having a structured thought technique that prioritizes common sense over feelings ensures that we first think through situations before performing.

Our first degree reaction to conditions and studies as humans is usually on an emotional degree. Any sensory enter we get hold of thru either of our five senses, sight, scent, hearing, touch or flavor is transmitted to the mind as a signal for interpretation. These signals are transmitted to the brain via the spinal code. The neuro sign first reaches the limbic machine part of the mind.

Emotional reactions originate from the limbic system for this reason the primary forestall for interpretation of any sensory enter is in the limbic system in which the sign is interpreted as an emotion before being exceeded on to the frontal lobe of the mind. The frontal lobe is charged with rational concept.

This organic pathway of transmission of sensory enter method that we're biologically stressed to first interpret situations on an emotional level earlier than decoding them rationally. This is why choices made in haste as reactions to feelings are frequently poorly concept out. Allowing emotions to persuade our idea process leads to terrible selections and ultimately the development of awful conduct.

By having sound intellectual fashions, we can set up a questioning manner that takes time to cautiously sift through information and apprehend the state of affairs before performing. We have all at one factor or some other given in to our feelings and made awful choices that we later regretted.

Negative and wonderful feelings are both detrimental to creating good decisions. When we're satisfied, we have a tendency to overlook possible pitfalls or bad results that may end result from our actions. While a advantageous body of mind is a superb element, it can intervene with our ability to be realistic and goal in choice making. Negative emotions have a tendency to elicit an destructive view of human beings and conditions.

Anger, unhappiness or tension are poor feelings that could pressure humans to adverse behavior and addictions in search of solace. Many addictions occur because of compulsive conduct which might be used as a shape of escape from bad emotions. Alcoholics, for example, are searching for solace within the numbing outcomes of the alcohol or the transient emotional excessive it presents. Failing to master your feelings can have disastrous consequences in non-public competence and within the capacity to narrate well with others.

Emotions and Mental Models

Emotions take place instinctively on a unconscious level and maximum of the time we aren't even aware about why we are feeling a certain manner. The introduction of emotion starts offevolved with the enjoy that we're exposed to. A physiological reaction based on the brain's interpretation of this revel in is then brought about. The very last step within the procedure is normally the behavioral expression of the emotion.

The human mind translates experiences as both positive or poor. When a bad incidence is perceived, the resulting physiological reaction is the manufacturing of strain hormones inclusive of adrenaline or cortisol. These stress hormones also are referred to as flight or fight hormones due to the fact they prepare the body to both fight or flee the threatening scenario. The resulting behavior in a threatening state of affairs is normally either aggression or flight.

In reviews that the mind perceives as high quality or worthwhile, the ensuing physiological response is the manufacturing of sense-desirable hormones. These include hormones which includes serotonin and oxytocin. These hormones bring about an ordinary feeling of nicely-being and happiness which is why they may be taken into consideration feel-desirable hormones. These hormones have an uplifting effect on our moods and could regularly put us in a superb frame of thoughts as a way to, in flip, affect how we behave, think and act.

The power of emotions over our lives is substantial and it's because of this that growing emotional intelligence is a prime basis ability for attaining personal boom. Understanding how feelings effect on our conduct and our relationships with others bureaucracy the premise of emotional intelligence. To attain emotional intelligence, we ought to enhance our capacities for self-awareness, self-regulation and relationship control.

Self-awareness is the capability to apprehend our feelings and recognize their affects on our conduct. Achieving self-focus calls for self-evaluation. It is from time to time tough to identify the feelings we're going thru and what triggers them. This is due to the fact emotions manifest at an instinctual stage and we hardly ever have the threat to identify their reason before they show up. Identifying our emotional triggers is the simplest manner we can be capable of alter them because this know-how offers us a deeper know-how of what's causing them.

Self-analysis is a essential step in achieving self-consciousness. When we analyze our emotions and the habits we develop as a result of these feelings we stand a higher danger of reaching behavior alternate. For instance, in case you recognise which you tend to drink alcohol whilst you are stressful, you may then are seeking to cope with the purpose of the anxiety in preference to trying to masks it.

Once you identify the trigger for the emotion it then becomes less difficult to address the motive of the dependancy. Similarly, while you may perceive what triggers your fine feelings you may cognizance greater on those conditions and on this manner create a happier life for yourself.

A loss of self-cognizance results in poor decision making, bad self-confidence and shortage of motivation. As human beings, we will always have strengths in some regions and weaknesses in others, the key to fulfillment is figuring out what our circle of competence is after which the use of this expertise to our benefit.

Self-regulation is an fundamental a part of emotional intelligence. It isn't enough to recognise what your emotions are and their associated triggers; we ought to additionally learn to manipulate them. Our natural intuition is to give in to our emotional impulses. However, when we allow feelings dominate our behavior, we lose the benefit of rational idea and reasoning. By reflecting on past stories and analyzing past consequences of conditions in which we used emotions to direct our actions, we are able to learn the result s of this emotionally driven behavior and learn how to keep our feelings in test.

Chapter 11: Mental Toughness Training

Mental durability. Google those words, and you'll locate hundreds of thousands of hits with anecdotes approximately Olympic athletes, West Point graduates, and military employees. You will even locate tales of ways human beings similar to you used this excessive-elegance skill to attain new heights in their own lives.

Mental sturdiness is the key ability that makes the distinction between a benched excessive college baseball pitcher going seasoned and in no way playing again. It's the difference among the Etsy store that just kind of peters out and one which turns into the owner's full dwelling. It's the distinction between your stagnancy and your glowing future. Another, less difficult phrase for mental sturdiness which you've probably heard before is that this: grit.

Determination. Perseverance. More than intelligence or genes or talent, that is the stuff that's been proven to set a success humans other than the rest. It's the drive to acquire long-time period goals, even when it's tough, or you don't feel adore it. Even when roadblocks upward push up to defeat you, with grit, you won't go into reverse.

At the very core of mental sturdiness is consistency. Once you create a aim, always striving toward it each day, one step at a time, is what's going to earn you grit. If you're an artist or need to be, that looks like growing something, even if it's small, every single day without failing. If you're an athlete, it looks as if showing up early to practice each unmarried time, completely focused and equipped to head, and by no means missing a workout. If you're a nurse, it looks like displaying up to your sufferers, even while you're worn-out, in any shape they want you to be.

The brilliant information about intellectual durability is this: you may have it. That voice for your head, that's been telling you someone else merits your desires due to the fact they're just more gifted or have better talents than you, is wrong. Talent and genetics can be completely overrun with the aid of one character who has the pressure and the self-discipline to consciousness tough on getting wherein they need to be. Anyone can gain mental toughness. That each person includes you.

Being mentally hard way, you'll be higher prepared for exchange. It approach you'll be greater high-quality below stress, greater effective during the workday, and harness extra emotional balance. It means you'll grow into the part of yourself that believes your happiness has not anything to do together with your outside world and everything to do along with your inner global.

Being mentally hard manner, you'll consciousness in your goals and goals as opposed to simply reacting to life as it comes. You'll be greater patient with the results because you could see simply the way you're getting there, and also you'll revel in a greater comfortable, content material countenance. All of this may be yours. Are you equipped to begin?

Training Yourself to be Mentally Tough

Step One: Know What You Want

To start with, you need to recognise what you need. You have that allows you to photo it surely in your mind. The first step is to make a clean, achievable intention. Define what being mentally hard looks as if in context for you.

If you need to smooth up your finances, maybe your mental longevity training for the week is making dinner every night time in place of succumbing to ordering takeout. If your goal is to be greater informed this year, commit to reading a e-book every week for the relaxation of the yr. If you need to work on sharpening your strength of will abilities, paintings your agenda so that you can healthy in an excellent dependancy, like meditating or walking. If you've been in reality bad recently approximately being present in your relationships, perhaps your first step is figuring out to depart your phone somewhere out of sight and spend 1/2 an hour along with your spouse and your children.

Notice how none of these duties seem to be mountains you couldn't climb. The task itself doesn't must be giant. The tough part is doing it always, every day, running at it even when you don't want to. There may be days you don't sense like cooking. Grit is grown by doing it while the incentive is at an rock bottom, simply because you understand you must.

When creating those dreams, keep in mind in which your roadblocks can be. Make positive the duties you create to accomplish your dreams are constructed into your habitual to emerge as a dependancy. When you don't want to or don't sense like showing up, engaging in your venture out of addiction will save you. Remember that being mentally difficult isn't about what feels exact. It's about sticking to the schedule no matter the way you experience about it. It's about being steady together with your behavior and your recurring to get in your purpose. That's what's going to set you apart. Every day when you entire your undertaking, make sure to have a good time your progress and your wins. Every step you're taking is getting you towards the individual you want to be.

Step Two: Tweak Your Self-Talk

Your mind is a effective machine, and it's continuously working. Whether you comprehend it or not, you assert 300 to at least one,000 phrases according to minute to yourself. What do they sound like? It might not appear like a large deal whilst you mutter, "Oh, that changed into silly," to your self after creating a mistake, or, "Yikes, that would've long gone better," whilst you bomb a presentation. But for Navy SEALs, self-communicate can suggest the difference among passing or failing. Welcome to the Pool Comp.

The Pool Competency Test is all about staying calm and nice whilst the whole thing round you threatens risk. Imagine this: you're underwater, decked out in scuba equipment. Everything is ordinary, in the surreal kind of manner the sector feels underwater. Suddenly, the system feeding oxygen in your mouth is ripped out, and the tube filling oxygen to that mouthpiece is tied in a knot.

If we went into this workout bloodless-turkey, with none education, our hearts would be racing. This is an issue of lifestyles and demise.

You ought to get your gadget back underneath control. But your hands are shaking, your mind is racing, and your coronary heart rate won't relax for an immediately. Panic sets in. Game over.

While our demanding situations might not be pool competency tests, that is a high-quality instance of the way education your thoughts to be tough can have an effect on how you behave, react, and get after your goals. The SEALs who were capable of think rationally and undoubtedly approximately their results at the same time as their lives had been at stake have been those who passed the exam, and additionally the ones who have the greatest intellectual durability.

Outside of probable saving your existence, research display that being high quality is really beneficial in many ways. Gratitude is validated to motive an growth in happiness, which isn't any wonder, considering gratitude is a willpower that makes us see the arena around us definitely.

Positivity also can be infectious for your relationships. A time period called social optimism states that simply believing that people will like you'll virtually make humans such as you extra. Optimism can gain you at paintings by way of growing extra opportunities for you, just because your high-quality mind-set is certain you may obtain them.

Tweaking yourself-talk towards positivity sounds smooth and instantly-ahead sufficient, however so lots of us have terrible self-speak already programmed into our brains as a habit. You must rewire your self to assume positively. Start with the aid of arising with truthful affirmations for moments of panic and tension. Pessimism has a tendency to tell you that awful matters remaining for all time, are universal, and suggest you're a terrible person. Here's an example.

Another candidate receives the task you've been working for the beyond 12 months to earn. Pessimism tells you this bad thing will ultimate forever. Your mind might say, "I'm in no way going to leave this office." Instead, tell yourself the truth: horrific matters skip. "I am going to get a higher function. It's simply no longer going on this time."

Similarly, pessimism will tell you that horrific things are widely wide-spread. You stroll out to the parking zone of the grocery keep and find that your vehicle's been hit, just in time to look at a youngster peel out of the parking zone and onto the adjoining road.

Fuming, you're in all likelihood questioning, "This could occur to me today! Things like this continually occur to me!" Instead of digging your self right into a rut of self-pity, alternate your mind. Bad matters have particular causes and don't just show up to you. Bad matters are not regular.

The remaining area your thoughts tends to wander while it's in hazard is responsible yourself. You ultimately got that new process you've been gunning for, however it's absolutely hard. Even in schooling, your new function calls for a number of attention and examine to recognize. Everything is unexpected. You might trudge home wondering, "I'm worthless. I can't do that." But is that the reality? No. The fact is which you're struggling with a new talent. You are not horrible at this process simply due to the fact you're suffering with it.

Another tool to struggle pessimism is to argue with yourself. If your brain is telling you something negative, use a mental model like Elon Musk's First Principles to dig to the foundation of the negativity. If the idea is, "I'll never be a very good dad," query why you believe you studied that. Is it due to the fact you don't have a good deal revel in in childcare? Is it due to the fact you'd want to be specific out of your dad and also you're no longer sure a way to try this?

Come up with a logical counter-argument, based totally in fact in preference to emotion (like your original poor notion probably is). Suddenly, "I'll in no way be a great dad," becomes, "I don't have an awful lot experience with youngsters, but if I work at it, I may have precise relationships with youngsters." If making a decision, your poor notion is one which desires to be countered even similarly, make it a point to create desires with a view to improve your counter-argument. Offer to babysit to your pals or a family member. Ask for help from a mother or a dad, and speak to them approximately your fears.

Often, positivity is a ability that's not noted as it's seen as less-than. People think about being nice as a bit of fluff to fill every other line on the "unique competencies" phase to your resume. The ever-faster, better, and more potent working monologue that's been floor into our brains says that any tool you can't use physically isn't worth using.

The reality about positivity, however, is that it's some thing a lot greater than we deliver it credit for. Some humans are naturally positive. It doesn't take a lot for them to look something beautiful in the wreckage. Others conflict with this talent. Either manner, strengthening it does greater advantage in your health, in your destiny work, and your relationships.

Conclusion

Life may be complex and it's easy to get beaten and burdened. There are continually choices to be made, troubles to be solved, and relationships to navigate. Sometimes, it can feel like your questioning is foggy, and also you want you had more readability. Other times, bad mind flood your thoughts and also you wish you may find a way to herald greater positivity. While you can't constantly alternate your surroundings or the situations you face, you can change your questioning. How? By increasing your wondering through intellectual fashions.

In this e book, you found out that intellectual fashions are distinct perspectives that affect the way you see the arena around you. We all have intellectual models evolved and informed through how we grew up and our stories, but they aren't always beneficial in every situation. That's why turning into familiar with as many models as feasible is essential. It's like including extra tools to a toolbox, so no matter what situation you discover yourself in, you can leaf through the container and find the tool that fits first-rate.

Mental fashions may be used for a variety of purposes. In this e book, we covered five: choice-making, seeing matters with more clarity, trouble-fixing, improving relationships, and wondering with more positivity. Many mental models have a couple of reason, like inversion, that is the process of thinking backwards from a selection or solution to a hassle. Other mental models we covered consist of:

• Paradox of preference - having too many alternatives can be paralyzing

• The "Why" model - breaking a confusing situation down through simply asking "why?"

• First ideas - breaking a hassle down to its most simple elements

• Hanlon's Razor - maximum of the time, humans aren't appearing out of malice, they're performing out of ignorance or carelessness

- The Pygmalion Effect - excessive expectations result in better effects

Rather than trying to exchange and manipulate what's around you, mental models pressure you to look inwardly and trade your self. That's all any of us simply have an influence on. If you need to improve your lifestyles and thinking, mastering more about the mental models you already own and mastering others is one of the high-quality paths to take.

www.ingramcontent.com/pod-product-compliance
Lightning Source LLC
Chambersburg PA
CBHW062136040426
42335CB00038B/1300